11.95

ABC OF
SEXUALLY TRANSMITTED DISEASES

ABC OF
SEXUALLY
TRANSMITTED DISEASES

SECOND EDITION

MICHAEL W ADLER MD FRCP

Professor of Genitourinary Medicine,
University College and Middlesex School of Medicine, London

with contributions from

IAN WELLER, DAVID GOLDMEIER

Published by the British Medical Association
Tavistock Square, London WC1H 9JR

First Edition 1984
Second Impression 1985
Third Impression (revised) 1986
Fourth Impression 1987
Fifth Impression 1988
Second Edition 1990
Second Impression 1992

British Library Cataloguing in Publication Data

Adler, Michael W.
    ABC of sexually transmitted diseases. – 2nd ed. – (ABC
series).
    1. Man. Sexually transmitted diseases
    I. Title   II. Weller, Ian   III. Goldmeier, David   IV.
Series
    616.951

ISBN 0–7279–0261–X

Typeset by
Latimer Trend & Company Ltd, Plymouth

Printed in England by Eyre & Spottiswoode Ltd, London and Margate

Contents

Page

A changing and growing problem   1

Urethral discharge: diagnosis   4

Urethral discharge: management   7

Vaginal discharge: diagnosis   9

Vaginal discharge: management   13

Complications of common genital infections and infections in other sites   17

Genital ulceration   22

Genital herpes   24

Viral hepatitis   IAN WELLER, *reader, Academic Department of Genitourinary Medicine, University College and Middlesex School of Medicine, London*   28

AIDS   IAN WELLER   32

Genital warts and molluscum contagiosum   40

Genital infestations   43

Genital skin and other conditions   46

Syphilis: clinical features   49

Syphilis: diagnosis and management   53

Pregnancy and the neonate   57

Psychological and sexual problems   DAVID GOLDMEIER, *consultant venereologist, St Mary's Hospital, London*   61

Methods of control   64

Index   68

A CHANGING AND GROWING PROBLEM

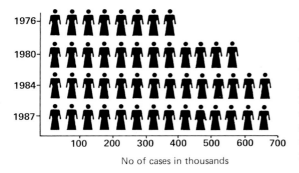

No of cases in thousands

The range of diseases spread by sexual activity continues to increase. In the United Kingdom the number of cases seen in sexually transmitted disease clinics (now known as departments of genitourinary medicine) has risen fourfold over the past 15 years and now amounts to nearly 700 000 new cases a year. For this reason sexually transmitted diseases need to be suspected and investigated in any patient who presents with what might at first look like a common clinical problem, such as a vaginal discharge, urinary tract infection, rash, or pelvic pain.

What are they?

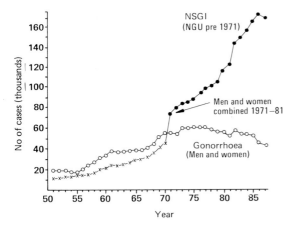

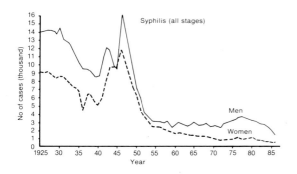

The commonest sexually transmitted diseases are non-specific genital infection and gonorrhoea. Until the middle 1970s there was a considerable increase in gonorrhoea in men and particularly women. There has been a recent decline. In women the rates are highest in those aged 20 to 24 years, but the largest increase has been among those under 20. Syphilis is not now a major problem, and the small rise in the incidence of syphilis (mainly primary and secondary) in the 1970s and early 1980s has occurred mainly in homosexuals. The recent decline is probably accounted for by the adoption of safer sex techniques among this group with the advent of HIV infection and AIDS.

Trichomoniasis, pediculosis pubis, genital warts, and herpes are common and are sexually transmitted. Warts now accounts for 84 000 cases and herpes for 18 000 and both are increasing more rapidly than other diseases. On the other hand, scabies and vaginal candidiasis are often diagnosed in sexually transmitted disease clinics, although they are not usually acquired sexually. Similarly, sexually transmitted hepatitis (A and B) is becoming more common, and recently those working in clinics have become aware of the possible sexual transmission of β haemolytic streptococci, cytomegalovirus, and enteric pathogens. The acquired immune deficiency syndrome with concomitant opportunistic infections and Kaposi's sarcoma in homosexuals is the most recent condition to be spread sexually.

Among a wide variety of other conditions presenting to clinics, and requiring specialist investigation and treatment, are urinary tract infections, pelvic inflammatory disease, dermatological and psychosexual problems as well as patients with a morbid fear of sexually transmitted diseases. Chancroid, granuloma inguinale, lymphogranuloma venereum, yaws, and pinta are now rare in Britain. Finally, many patients (27% of the total cases) seek reassurance, require simple counselling or advice, and want check ups; all need to be investigated.

A changing and growing problem

Why have they increased?

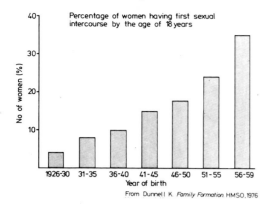

Percentage of women having first sexual intercourse by the age of 18 years

From Dunnell K. *Family Formation.* HMSO, 1976

Like many other medicosocial conditions—for example, suicide, alcoholism, cancer, and heart disease—the explanation for the increase in the sexually transmitted diseases is multifactorial.

The age of sexual maturity has decreased, the age at which people have sexual intercourse for the first time is lower, and more people have premarital sexual intercourse than previously. None of these indicate promiscuity, but it must be a factor. Also, the increasing use of the oral contraceptive pill and intrauterine devices has removed the protective effect of barrier techniques such as the sheath.

Because of the greatly improved service offered by the clinics and their ability to trace sexual contacts more people are seeking treatment who may not have previously done so. Thus how much of the increase in the number of recorded cases reflects a real or apparent trend is unknown.

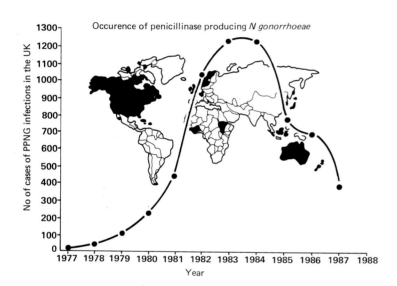

Occurence of penicillinase producing *N gonorrhoeae*

Since populations are now more mobile nationally and internationally certain groups (tourists, professional travellers, members of the armed forces, immigrants) are at risk. They are separated from their families and social restraints and are more likely to have sexual contact outside a stable relationship.

Over the years the partial resistance of the gonococcus to penicillin has increased in many countries so that higher and higher curative doses have had to be used. More worrying than this is the recent emergence of penicillin resistant strains of *Neisseria gonorrhoeae*. The number of cases of gonorrhoea in the United Kingdom due to these penicillinase producing strains initially doubled each year from 1977 until 1983 but has recently declined.

The final factor in the increasing incidence is the lack of resources for both good treatment facilities and coordinated research. Many countries still do not accept the importance of an open access, free service for sexually transmitted diseases, and even those countries with this facility often provide it in poor and old premises.

How do they present?

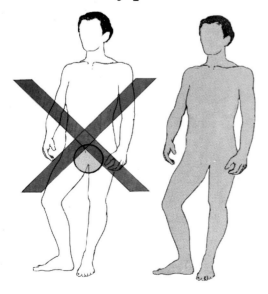

The three commonest presenting symptoms are urethral discharge, genital ulceration, and vaginal discharge with or without vulval irritation. The descriptions in later chapters of the many diseases that may be spread sexually will show that patients may present with other symptoms (rash, dysuria, jaundice, arthralgia, rectal discharge). Additionally, several diseases may present initially with complications (abdominal or scrotal pain, urinary retention). Since they may affect any system in the body they should not be regarded solely as diseases of the genitals. Finally, the diseases are not always acute; many chronic conditions of the genital tract require long term management—for example, pelvic pain, recurrent herpes genitalis, and vaginal candidiasis.

How should they be managed?

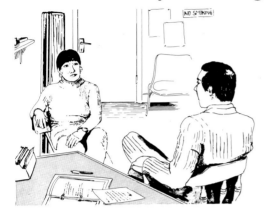

The most important aspects of management are accurate diagnosis and effective treatment. Diagnosis needs time and skill in taking a detailed sexual history from both the patient and his or her sexual contacts and in carrying out a comprehensive physical examination. But above all microbiological and serological facilities are essential initially and at follow up for all patients to differentiate between the various diseases, exclude more than one occurring at a time, and identify asymptomatic disease. Some doctors have the facilities to perform some microbiological tests in their surgeries, but if not referral to a clinic is strongly advised. These clinics now have a much more relaxed image and offer the patient a chance to seek help and advice with complete confidence and confidentiality.

To prevent the spread of sexually transmitted diseases treatment must be effective and be seen to be effective. This means selecting the correct drug for the disease, carefully monitoring its administration, and carrying out regular follow up microbiological tests. The patient's sexual contacts must be traced so that they can be treated and thus prevent the disease from spreading further. The doctor may also play an important part in controlling the diseases by advising patients how best to avoid them, to recognise them, and to have them treated and by offering the opportunity for routine check ups for those who have put themselves at risk or who simply want reassurance. All of these facilities are offered within departments of genitourinary medicine.

The workload of specialists in genitourinary medicine is continually increasing. Firstly, this is due to the realisation over the years that more and more diseases may be spread sexually, a point vividly illustrated recently by the epidemic of HIV infection and AIDS. Secondly, it is appreciated that other acute and chronic non-sexually acquired conditions are being managed in clinics. Genitourinary medicine is now a specialty in its own right, offering total care of people with a wide variety of conditions. The increased breadth of the specialty, and the knowledge that many patients seen in clinics do not have a sexually transmitted disease, have helped to reduce the stigma attached to clinics and should be of help to general practitioners, gynaecologists, and others wishing to refer patients for specialist advice.

Management
Sexual history
Physical examination
Microbiology
Serology
Tracing sexual contacts
Education
Reassurance
Follow up

Sexually transmitted diseases in the United Kingdom for 1987
(Figures are numbers of cases)

Non-specific genital infection	146 636	Other treponemal diseases	539
Genital warts	84 615	Molluscum contagiosum	3 478
Candidiasis	65 597	Chancroid	41
Gonorrhoea	28 568	Granuloma inguinale	28
Genital herpes	17 966	Lymphogranuloma venereum	18
Trichomoniasis	11 520	Other conditions: Not requiring treatment	181 385
Pediculosis pubis	7 836	Requiring treatment	121 545
Syphilis	1 730		
Scabies	1 501		
		Total	673 003

Micro-organisms that can be sexually transmitted

Bacteria:
  Chlamydia trachomatis
  Neisseria gonorrhoeae
  Gardnerella vaginalis
  Treponema pallidum
  Group B haemolytic streptococcus
  Haemophilus ducreyi
  Calymmatobacterium granulomatis
  Shigella species
Mycoplasmas:
  Ureaplasma urealyticum
  Mycoplasma hominis
Parasites:
  Sarcoptes scabiei
  Phthirus pubis

Viruses:
  Herpes simplex virus types 1 and 2
  Wart virus (papillomavirus)
  Molluscum contagiosum virus (poxvirus)
  Hepatitis A and B virus
  Cytomegalovirus
  Human immunodeficiency virus 1 and 2
Protozoa:
  Entamoeba histolytica
  Giardia lamblia
  Trichomonas vaginalis
Fungi:
  Candida albicans

URETHRAL DISCHARGE: DIAGNOSIS

The commonest presenting symptom
of a sexually transmitted disease
in men

A urethral discharge is the commonest presenting symptom of a sexually transmitted disease in men. A few discharges may be physiological but most are pathological; most of those seen by both general practitioners and specialists are pathological.

Causes

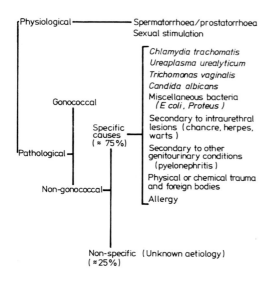

Broadly, pathological discharges are either gonococcal, due to infection with *Neisseria gonorrhoeae*, or non-gonococcal. The commonest cause of non-gonococcal urethritis is *Chlamydia trachomatis*, but it may also be due to infection with *Ureaplasma urealyticum*, *Trichomonas vaginalis*, or *Candida albicans* and sometimes to intraurethral lesions such as herpes genitalis, warts, or a syphilitic chancre. All these infections are acquired sexually. Rarely, pyelonephritis or a urinary tract infection may produce a urethral discharge. Attempts at intraurethral self medication with chemicals may cause a discharge, as may trauma from the use of sexual aids or the self inflicted lesions of dermatitis artefacta.

In about a quarter of cases of non-gonococcal urethritis no cause or infective agent may be identifed, and these may be designated as true non-specific urethritis. Usually these discharges are assumed to be caused by a sexually transmitted infection which requires treatment.

Small amounts of clear or mucoid urethral discharge after sexual intercourse are probably the result of sexual stimulation. In the absence of sexual arousal the discharge may be due to spermatorrhoea or prostatorrhoea, both of which may be noticed at urination or defecation.

Taking a history

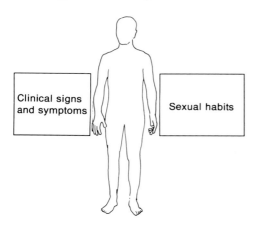

An accurate history must be taken, particularly of the clinical features and sexual factors, and a physical examination and full microbiological tests performed.

Clinical features—When a patient complains of a discharge it is important to identify its site. Uncircumcised men may develop a subpreputial infection (for example, herpetic or candidal) or disease (for example, inflammation from smegma or trauma, skin disorders, or malignancy) but find it difficult to pinpoint the exact source of the discharge. The patient may describe the colour and quantity of the discharge as yellow, white, clear, profuse, scanty, or a combination of these. Such descriptions give little indication of the type of infective agent present. Likewise, the fact that the incubation period of gonorrhoea (two to five days) is often shorter than for chlamydial or other types of non-gonococcal infection (seven to 14 days) should not be used to make a non-microbiological clinical diagnosis. Five to 10% of patients with gonococcal or non-gonococcal urethritis have no symptoms.

Sexual factors—Details of the number and type of sexual contact in the previous four weeks and whether or not the partner has symptoms or has been treated recently must be determined. If the patient is homosexual it is necessary to know which anatomical sites have been exposed to risk—for example, the rectum or the throat as well as the urethra or a combination of all three. More than one site may be affected, and appropriate tests on samples from the rectum, throat or both—as well as from the urethra—may be needed. Because of the development of strains of *N gonorrhoeae* that are resistant to penicillin details of sexual contact in other countries must be obtained. In all cases contact tracing of sexual contacts needs to be carried out to determine the source of the infection and the people who may in turn have been infected by the patient.

Sexual history
Homosexual or heterosexual
Number of partners
Symptoms in partner(s)
Overseas contact
Sites of contact

Physical examination

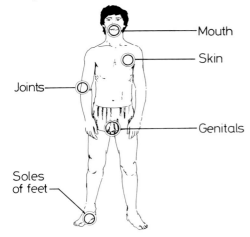

The penis should be thoroughly examined, particularly with the prepuce retracted, as should the scrotum and its contents, the pubic hair and surrounding skin, and the perianal area. The physical examination should not be limited to the genitals since with a "fly button" approach important information may be missed. A thorough general physical examination is needed to exclude possible complications of gonorrhoea or non-gonococcal infection. Often patients have more than one sexually transmitted disease at a time, and these may be missed unless the patient is comprehensively examined. Particular attention should be paid to the skin, soles of the feet, mouth, and joints. The need to undertake a detailed physical examination is illustrated by HIV infection and AIDS, which can present in virtually any system of the body.

A specimen of urethral discharge must be collected for Gram staining and microscopical examination. The slides may be stained immediately and a presumptive diagnosis of gonococcal or non-gonococcal urethritis made. Gonorrhoea will be confirmed by the presence of Gram negative intracellular diplococci, whereas non-gonococcal urethritis will be confirmed by their absence but the presence of ≥5 polymorphonuclear leucocytes per high power field (×1000 magnification). *C trachomatis* cannot, however, be identified by direct microscopy.

T vaginalis is not a common cause of urethral discharge and is probably worth looking for only in patients with chronic urethritis and those whose female sexual contacts already have trichomoniasis. A specimen of discharge is placed on a slide (with one drop of saline), a coverslip added, and examined without staining under the microscope with dark ground illumination.

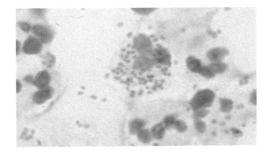

Culture

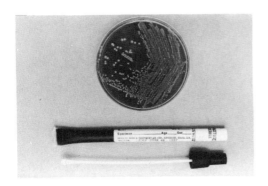

As up to 10% of cases of gonorrhoea may be missed if microscopy alone forms the basis of diagnosis specimens of urethral discharge should ideally be cultured for *N gonorrhoeae*. The discharge may be plated directly on to a selective medium—for example, Thayer-Martin or modified New York City medium—which has added antibiotics to suppress overgrowth by other micro-organisms. The plates are incubated at 37°C in an enriched carbon dioxide environment (5–10%) for 48 hours in candle extinction jars or a carbon dioxide incubator. If a transport medium is needed either Stuart's or Amies's may be used, but specimens must reach the laboratory for plating out (as above) within 24 hours. Confirmatory tests, such as oxidase reaction, sugar fermentation, or immunofluorescence on suspected cultures help to distinguish *N gonorrhoeae* from other organisms.

Unfortunately, most laboratories supporting departments of genitourinary medicine cannot provide a routine culture service for *C trachomatis*, although 30-50% of men with non-gonococcal urethritis may have a chlamydial infection. The advent of newer technology will

Urethral discharge: diagnosis

allow the detection of chlamydial antigen without the need for cell culture. These techniques—for example, immunofluorescence and enzyme immunoassay—use both polyclonal and monoclonal antibodies.

Blood and urine tests

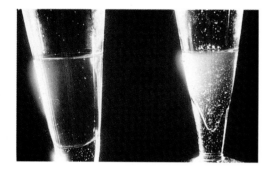

A urine sample should be collected. In the two glass urine test the patient is asked to pass about 60–120 ml into the first glass (first voided urine) and the remainder of his specimen into the second. The presence of threads or specks of pus and a hazy appearance which is not due to phosphates—that is, it does not clear after 5–10% acetic acid has been added—in the first glass confirms anterior urethritis. This test may easily be carried out by the general practitioner before referral and will help to differentiate an anterior from a posterior urethritis, a cystitis, or a nephritis (hazy urine with thread in both glasses). The referring practitioner should advise the patient to hold his urine for at least four hours before attending the clinic; this allows for the discharge to collect within the urethra. Some patients who give a history of discharge have no evidence of this when examined. In these cases it may be worth while repeating the investigations after the patient has held his urine overnight.

Although the gonococcal complement fixation test is of no use in the diagnosis of gonorrhoea blood samples should be collected from all patients to exclude concurrent infection with syphilis.

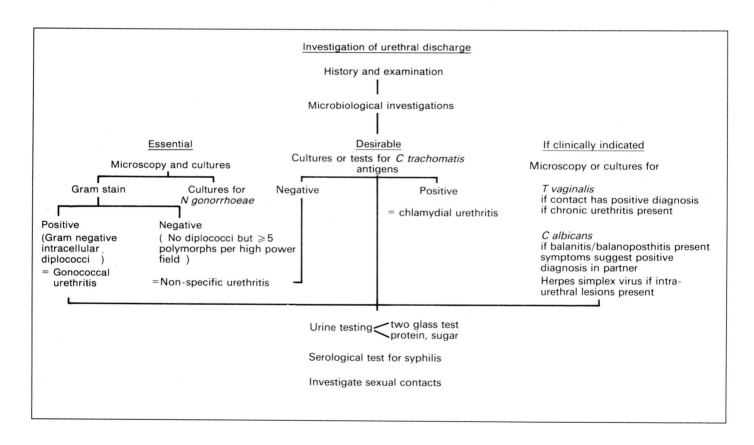

URETHRAL DISCHARGE: MANAGEMENT

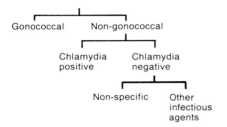

Gonococcal urethritis

Chemotherapy
Aqueous procaine penicillin Benzylpenicillin Ampicillin Amoxycillin
<u>If allergic to penicillin:</u> Spectinomycin Tetracycline Co-trimoxazole Cefuroxime

Since the treatment of a gonococcal urethritis differs fundamentally from that for non-gonococcal urethritis an accurate microbiological diagnosis is essential, as are repeated microbiological tests at follow up. For this reason, and because of the need to exclude concurrent infections and trace sexual contacts, many doctors may prefer their patients to attend their local department of genitourinary medicine after initial physical examination and investigation and investigations in the surgery (see box).

Chemotherapy—Penicillin is the drug of choice and may be given either intramuscularly as aqueous procaine penicillin 2·4 MU preceded by probenecid 1 g orally or as 5 MU of benzylpenicillin in 8 ml of 0·5% lignocaine with probenecid 1 g or by mouth as ampicillin 3–3·5 g in a single dose with probenecid 1 g. Other oral preparations, such as amoxycillin 3 g plus probenecid, may be used but do not offer higher cure rates than ampicillin and are more expensive.

If the patient is allergic to penicillin then spectinomycin 2 g intramuscularly, tetracycline 500 mg by mouth every six hours for five days, co-trimoxazole four tablets by mouth twice daily for two days, or ciprofloxacin 250 mg immediately by mouth may be given. Neither tetracycline nor co-trimoxazole is as effective as penicillin, but since co-trimoxazole is not treponemicidal it may be given to those patients being investigated for suspected syphilis. These regimens are suggested for use only in the United Kingdom. Regimens in other countries will depend on the sensitivities of the gonococcus, the availability of antibiotics, and the ability to follow up the patient after treatment. Since patients may not return some countries advocate the use of tetracycline in the treatment of gonorrhoea since it will eradicate *N gonorrhoeae* as well as concurrent infection with *Chlamydia trachomatis*. Another approach is to give a course of oxytetracycline 500 mg four times a day for seven days in combination with penicillin, so eradicating possible chlamydial infection.

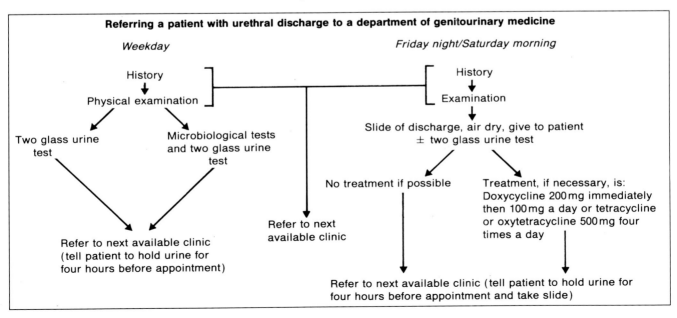

Urethral discharge: management

Follow up—Within three to seven days after treatment the patient should have further microbiological tests of cure (smears and cultures) carried out and if satisfactory again if possible after a further week. He should be advised to abstain from further sexual contact until this final follow up visit. All sexual contacts should be encouraged to attend a clinic or their general practitioner for investigation and treatment. Serological tests for syphilis should be carried out for all patients after three months, as the initial investigations may have become positive by the end of the full incubation period of this condition.

Treatment failure

Treatment failure

Reinfection:

    Penicillin

Reistant infections:

    Spectinomycin

    Cefuroxime

Postgonococcal urethritis:

    Tetracycline

If patients with a gonococcal urethritis do not respond to penicillin and still harbour *N gonorrhoeae* two possibilities need to be considered: reinfection or infection with a penicillinase producing strain of *N gonorrhoeae*. Reinfection needs further treatment with penicillin whereas an infection due to a resistant strain of *N gonorrhoeae* must be treated with spectinomycin 2 g intramuscularly or cefuroxime 1·5 g intramuscularly with probenecid 1 g orally.

Some patients (25–50%) develop a postgonococcal urethritis after treatment with penicillin. It is not unusual at the first follow up visit to find a residual urethritis with polymorphonuclear leucocytes on the Gram stained smear and evidence of pyuria in the first glass of urine. Postgonococcal urethritis should not, therefore, be diagnosed until two weeks after the original infection has been treated. Culture will by definition be negative for *N gonorrhoeae*. Postgonococcal urethritis is caused by *C trachomatis* in 80% of cases. Tetracycline 500 mg should be given every six hours for seven days or doxycycline 100 mg twice a day for seven days. If the discharge persists the same regimen should be continued for a further seven days.

Non-gonococcal urethritis

Chemotherapy

Tetracycline

Oxytetracycline

Triple tetracycline

Doxycycline

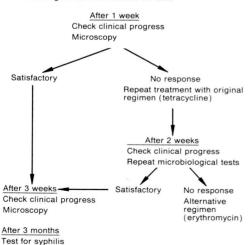

Advice and follow up

Avoid sexual intercourse and milk products
Investigate and treat sexual contacts

After 1 week
Check clinical progress
Microscopy

Satisfactory

No response
Repeat treatment with original
regimen (tetracycline)

After 2 weeks
Check clinical progress
Repeat microbiological tests

Satisfactory

No response
Alternative
regimen
(erythromycin)

After 3 weeks
Check clinical progress
Microscopy

After 3 months
Test for syphilis

Chemotherapy—Fortunately, the same treatment regimen is effective in both chlamydia positive and chlamydia negative non-gonococcal urethritis. The tetracyclines are the antibiotic of first choice, usually tetracycline or oxytetracycline, 500 mg six hourly for seven days. Doxycycline 100 mg twice a day also for seven days is as effective but more expensive. The patient should be advised to avoid sexual intercourse and milk products.

Follow up—Even though a one week course of a tetracycline is effective in curing both chlamydia positive and chlamydia negative non-gonococcal urethritis, patient compliance and drug absorption have to be perfect for this to occur. Thus after one week of treatment the patient should be seen so that compliance, side effects, and clinical progress can be assessed. Microscopy should also be carried out and if satisfactory and possible finally again two weeks later (three weeks after the initial diagnosis and treatment). If the urethritis has not responded after one week of treatment a further week's treatment must be given. If the discharge still persists after 14 days' treatment erythromycin stearate 500 mg should be given 12 hourly for 14 days. The sexual contacts of all patients undergoing treatment must be investigated and treated. Unfortunately, this is sometimes overlooked until it becomes clear that the patient with persistent infection is being reinfected by his partner(s). Finally, a patient with non-gonococcal urethritis should be investigated for syphilis after three months.

On occasions the urethritis becomes chronic and further investigations—for example, of the prostate—will be needed. All too often, however, these patients are not suffering from infective urethritis but have become anxious self examiners and "squeezers," a condition reinforced by inexperienced doctors who treat the microscope slide and not the whole patient.

Other infective agents only rarely give rise to a urethral discharge; those due to *T vaginalis*, *C albicans*, warts, herpes simplex virus, syphilitic chancre, and trauma are covered in later chapters.

VAGINAL DISCHARGE: DIAGNOSIS

Vaginal discharge is a common presenting symptom seen by general practitioners, gynaecologists, and those working in family planning clinics and departments of genitourinary medicine. As with urethral discharge, vaginal discharge may be either physiological or pathological in origin. It is difficult to know what proportion of discharges belong to either category since there have been few community based prevalence studies.

Physiological causes—Vaginal discharge is a continuum, and as such the concept of normality does not exist. Some patients have a copious discharge, others none or little. Only the patient can, therefore, determine what is her own normal experience. It is worthwhile reminding patients that a normal vaginal discharge may increase and be noticed only premenstrually, at the time of ovulation, or when using the contraceptive pill or an intrauterine device. Non-pathological lesions on the cervix such as ectropion can cause a discharge.

Pathological (infective) causes—The commonest organism giving rise to an infective pathological vaginal discharge is *Candida albicans*. Other causes of this symptom include vaginal infections with *Trichomonas vaginalis, Gardnerella vaginalis*, and anaerobic organisms, and cervical infections with *Neisseria gonorrhoea* and *Chlamydia trachomatis*. Cervical lesions due to herpes, warts, and a syphilitic chancre may also cause a discharge. There is some doubt about whether *Ureaplasma urealyticum* and haemolytic streptococci do cause a vaginal discharge, and the discharge of the rare toxic shock syndrome is usually coincidental and overshadowed by the patient's general condition.

Pathological (non-infective) causes—Localised cervical lesions such as polyps and neoplasms may present with a vaginal discharge. It is surprising what may be retained in the vagina without the patient's knowledge: tampons and the occasional condom are common, but cloves of garlic have also been found. Trauma may be caused by sexual aids and irritant substances.

Pathological causes

Infective:
  Candida albicans
  Trichomonas vaginalis
  Gardnerella vaginalis
  Anaerobic organisms
  Chlamydia trachomatis
  Neisseria gonorrhoeae
  Cervical herpes genitalis
  Cervical warts
  Syphilitic chancre
  Toxic shock syndrome
    (*? Staphylococcus aureus*)
  Mycoplasmas
  β haemolytic streptococci
Non-infective:
  Cervical ectropion
  Cervical polyp(s)
  Neoplasm
  Retained products
    (tampon, postabortion, postnatal)
  Trauma
  Allergy

History

As with urethral discharge, a careful history, physical examination, and microbiological tests are essential to establish an accurate diagnosis and to exclude a sexually acquired infection.

Certain points in the clinical history suggest that a sexually transmitted disease is a possibility—such as the development of symptoms after a recent change of sexual partner or recent multiple sexual contacts. To be certain of avoiding contracting a sexually transmitted disease both partners need to be monogamous. Further points that should make the doctor suspect a sexually transmitted disease are symptoms in the patient that are recurrent or persistent and symptoms in her sexual partner. A urethral discharge in a woman's partner makes it highly likely that her symptoms are due to a sexually transmitted infection. Irritation, soreness, and redness of her partner's penis after sexual contact suggests infection with *Candida albicans*. Finally, the patient should be asked about any other symptoms that suggest complications of a sexually transmitted disease—for example, abdominal pain, rash, arthralgia, dyspareunia, or altered menstruation.

High risk profile

Partner change
Multiple contacts
Recurrent symptoms
Symptoms in partner
General symptoms:

  Abdominal pain
  Menstrual problems
  Rash
  Dyspareunia
  Arthralgia

Vaginal discharge: diagnosis

Neither the patient's symptoms nor a subjective description of the colour and quality of the discharge are of much value in reaching an accurate diagnosis. Even more so than in men genitourinary symptoms in women are a poor guide to the exact nature of the condition.

Physical and laboratory investigations

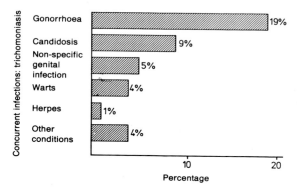

If a sexually transmitted disease is suspected from the clinical and sexual history the patient should be examined fully to exclude possible complications and coincidental abnormalities. Once the physical examination has been carried out local genital examination and tests should be undertaken. As with the symptoms, the physical signs and macroscopic appearance of a vaginal discharge do not help in making an accurate diagnosis. For instance, to rely on the suggestion that the discharge of vaginal candidiasis is thick, curdy, and white will result in the wrong diagnosis in most instances. Similarly, no reliance should be placed on the supposed association between a frothy greenish discharge and trichomoniasis.

Infection can be diagnosed accurately only after microbiological tests have been carried out on samples from the appropriate anatomical sites. Women attending departments of genitourinary medicine have tests performed routinely to establish or exclude a diagnosis of candidiasis, trichomoniasis, gonorrhoea, and often *Chlamydia trachomatis* infection. So that samples may be obtained from the appropriate sites a speculum should be passed to visualise accurately the cervix, posterior fornix, and the vagina. The reason these tests are performed routinely is because sexually transmitted diseases may occur concurrently. In clinics one fifth of the cases of trichomoniasis are associated with gonorrhoea. Many authorities do not consider that candidiasis is sexually transmitted, but despite this it is associated with other sexually acquired conditions in a third of cases.

Candida albicans may be excluded by microscopy of a Gram stained smear and by culture of material from the vaginal wall. Both cells and mycelia stain Gram positive. Since some cases may be missed when microscopy alone is relied on cultures should be carried out to confirm the diagnosis or they may be used alone without microscopy. Traditionally, cultures are plated on Sabouraud's medium and incubated at 37°C for 48 hours; Stuart's or Amies's transport medium may be used when necessary. Other yeasts—for example, *Torulopsis glabrata*—also occasionally inhabit the female genital tract and grow on culture. Definitive differentiation may be achieved only by additional tests. *Trichomonas vaginalis* is usually best isolated from the posterior fornix, and a wet preparation using a drop of saline should be examined immediately by dark ground microscopy. Though the diagnosis may be confirmed by culture, microscopy alone is extremely reliable. The specimen of discharge must be placed directly into Feinberg–Whittington medium and incubated for 48 hours at 37°C or sent to the laboratories in Stuart's or Amies's transport media.

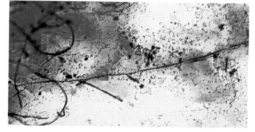

Mycelia

Gonorrhoea is an infection of mucous membranes, and since the vagina is lined with stratified squamous epithelium a high vaginal swab is not the best method of sampling in diagnosing this condition. The most productive sites for isolating the gonococcus are the endocervix and the urethra. Specimens should be taken from both sites, Gram stained, and cultured. As with specimens of urethral discharge the culture material may be put into a suitable transport medium (for example, Stuart's) or plated directly and incubated. Gram stained microscopy for *Neisseria gonorrhoeae* in women is unreliable. Reliance on this alone results in about a half of cases being missed. All women in whom gonorrhoea is suspected should therefore have cultures performed in addition to microscopy. One set of smears and cultures should detect 90% of cases. This figure may be increased by repeat testing and by sampling other sites.

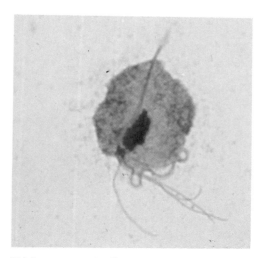

Trichomonas vaginalis

Gonorrhoea: diagnosis by site of infection

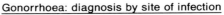

Gonorrhoea

Samples from:	Microscopy (Gram stained smear)
Urethra	
Endocervix	Culture
Rectum (for sexual contacts of men with gonorrhoea)	

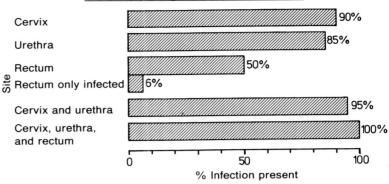

Gonorrhoea: diagnosis by site of infection

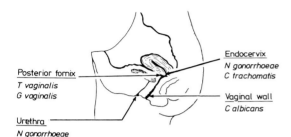

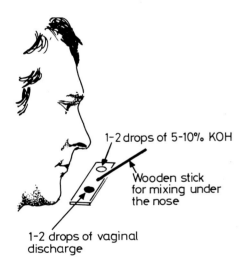

1-2 drops of 5-10% KOH

Wooden stick for mixing under the nose

1-2 drops of vaginal discharge

The gonococcus may be isolated from the rectum in women with gonorrhoea in about 6% of cases in which it is not found in the conventional sites, the cervix and urethra. Proctitis arises more often by autoinoculation from vaginal discharge than from anal intercourse. For this reason all women who are contacts of men with gonorrhoea should have rectal tests carried out in the hope of increasing the chances of isolating the gonococcus.

C trachomatis is now known to be an important sexually transmitted agent which often causes asymptomatic infections and may occur concurrently with other sexually acquired agents, in particular *N gonorrhoeae*. Unfortunately, facilities do not yet exist for identifying this micro-organism in all laboratories supporting departments of genitourinary medicine. If they do an endocervical specimen should be taken for *C trachomatis* in any woman attending a clinic. If only limited microbiological services are available tests should be limited to women who will not receive treatment with antichlamydial drugs (patients with gonorrhoea and unknown contact histories) and in those presenting with a complication—for example, pelvic inflammatory disease.

Vaginal discharge can also occur as a result of anaerobic vaginosis/non-specific vaginitis. Certain clinical and diagnostic features seem to be associated with this infection: a fishy smelling discharge, which is particularly noticeable after sexual intercourse; the presence of clue cells (bacteria attached to vaginal epithelial cells) in a drop of infected discharge mixed with saline and viewed under the microscope; a pH of the vaginal discharge ≥ 5 (easily measured by pH paper); and a positive result on the amine test. This test is performed by adding one to two drops of discharge and 5–10% potassium hydroxide together on a glass slide. If a fishy ammoniacal odour is released the result is positive. A similar smell may be obtained when *T vaginalis* or spermatozoa are present in the vaginal discharge. *Gardnerella vaginalis* and a mixture of anaerobes—for example, *Bacteroides* spp, peptococci, peptostreptococci, mobiluncus—are usually found in high concentrations in patients with bacterial vaginosis. Diagnosis is made on the above criteria without the need for culture.

Finally, all patients should have serological tests for syphilis carried out to exclude this as a concurrent infection, their urine tested for protein and glucose, and cervical cytology if not performed in the previous year.

Isolation rate for *C trachomatis*	
Gonorrhoea contacts	30-60%
Non-gonococcal urethritis contacts	30-35%
Attending GUM clinics (excluding above groups)	2-17%
Attending family planning/well women clinics	2-7%

Vaginal discharge: diagnosis

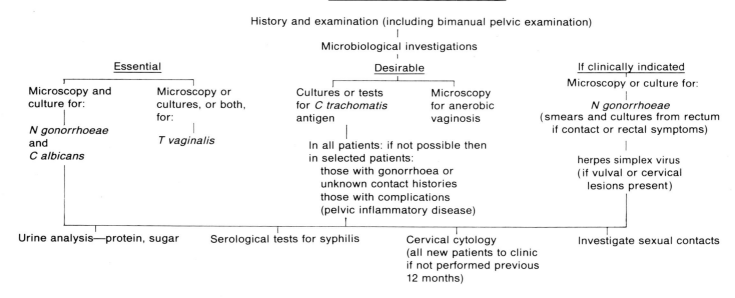

Investigation of vaginal discharge

History and examination (including bimanual pelvic examination)

Microbiological investigations

Essential

Microscopy and culture for:

N gonorrhoeae and *C albicans*

Microscopy or cultures, or both, for:

T vaginalis

Desirable

Cultures or tests for *C trachomatis* antigen

In all patients: if not possible then in selected patients:
    those with gonorrhoea or unknown contact histories
    those with complications (pelvic inflammatory disease)

Microscopy for anerobic vaginosis

If clinically indicated

Microscopy or culture for:

N gonorrhoeae (smears and cultures from rectum if contact or rectal symptoms)

herpes simplex virus (if vulval or cervical lesions present)

Urine analysis—protein, sugar   Serological tests for syphilis   Cervical cytology (all new patients to clinic if not performed previous 12 months)   Investigate sexual contacts

VAGINAL DISCHARGE: MANAGEMENT

Vaginal candidiasis

Management

Vaginal pessaries:

  Nystatin

  Clotrimazole

  Miconazole

  Econazole

Genital hygiene:

  Clean

  Dry

  Avoid trauma or irritation

Assess clinical and microbiological

  response

Treat other infections/conditions

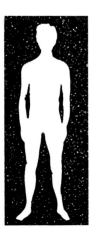

See male contacts if:

They have symptoms

Their partner has
recurrences

Despite the introduction of a new oral antifungal agent (ketoconazole) the cornerstone of the treatment of vaginal candidiasis is still local pessaries. Straightforward nystatin pessaries (two of 100 000 units each inserted into the vagina at night for two weeks) have stood the test of time. Their rather dry brittle consistency and the length of treatment, however, often raise doubts about patient acceptability and compliance. More recently introduced imidazole preparations (clotrimazole, miconazole, econazole) are softer and need only be prescribed for shorter periods—for example, clotrimazole pessaries 500 mg once at night or 200 mg nightly for three days. Vulval irritation may be relieved by local nystatin or clotrimazole cream applied twice a day.

The condition may recur, but recurrence is also often preventable and it is always worth explaining simple methods of genital hygiene and the possible precipitating factors to the patient at the time of her initial attack, since this may help the condition to resolve and prevent recurrences. The patient should be advised to keep the genital area clean, dry, and untraumatised, ideally by not wearing nylon pants, tights, or jeans. Since autoinfection from the bowel may occur cleaning with toilet paper should be in a backwards direction.

Predisposing factors—Trauma to the vaginal mucosa may predispose to infection and may occur during intercourse or when vaginal deodorants, perfumed soaps, and bubble baths are used. The patient may require additional lubrication with K-Y jelly during sexual intercourse. Pregnancy, antibiotics, corticosteroid and immunosuppressive treatment, diabetes, orogenital contact, and the presence of other sexually transmitted diseases have all been implicated in both initial and recurrent disease. The sexual partner may occasionally be the source of infection and reinfection.

Follow up—If possible patients should be seen at least once after treatment to assess the clinical and microbiological response and so that any other treatment may be started if additional sexually acquired infections have been identified in the laboratory after the initial set of tests at first consultation.

Treatment of relapsing infection—A relapse shortly after initial treatment needs a longer course of treatment—for example, if clotrimazole is used 100 mg should be given daily for 12 days. If this regimen fails an increased dose of 200 mg daily should be given for 12 days. Controversy exists about whether this should be combined with oral nystatin 500 000 units every eight hours for one to two weeks to combat possible reinfection from the bowel since recolonisation occurs rapidly after treatment has been stopped. Prophylactic treatment may be tried with clotrimazole 500 mg once a week or month for two to three months.

Sexual contacts—Candidiasis is not usually sexually transmitted but male contacts should be seen, firstly, if they have symptoms and, secondly, if the woman is having repeated recurrences. The man should be thoroughly investigated, as was his female partner, to make sure that he has no concurrent sexually transmitted disease, since this is likely to predispose to candidal infection. Candidal balanitis is treated with saline bathing and application of nystatin or clotrimazole cream.

Ketoconazole is expensive, produces side effects, and has not been fully assessed for use in vaginal candidiasis. At present it is best reserved for chronic mucocutaneous candidiasis and possibly superficial mycoses.

Trichomoniasis

Management

Clinical history

Confirm by microbiological diagnosis

Treat with metronidazole, avoid alcohol

Follow up:

    Assess microbiological response
    Repeat treatment if necessary

Investigate and treat sexual contacts

Infestation with *Trichomonas vaginalis* should be treated with metronidazole 400 mg twice daily for five days or a single dose of metronidazole or nimorazole 2 g. The patient should be warned of the possible disulfiram like (Antabuse) effect of these drugs in association with alcohol. Unless patients are warned they quite logically give up the tablets rather than the alcohol. Patients should be followed up at least once for microbiological tests of cure after treatment, and so that any other infections detected may be treated. Patients not responding to treatment should be given metronidazole 800 mg every 12 hours for five days. Continued failure usually indicates that (*a*) the patient is being reinfected by her sexual partner; (*b*) she is not complying with the medication; (*c*) the drug is not being absorbed; or (*d*) it is being inhibited locally by vaginal bacteria. Sometimes patients need to be admitted to hospital for supervision of treatment. The serum concentrations of metronidazole may be estimated and vaginal bacteria inhibiting the action of the drug detected in patients who fail to respond to treatment but are complying and not being reinfected.

Treatment failure

Reinfection

Non-compliance

Poor absorption

Inhibition by vaginal bacteria

Treatment in pregnancy—Laboratory studies on animals have suggested that massive doses of metronidazole are teratogenic, even though this effect has not been reported in humans. It is therefore probably unwise to use it in the first trimester of pregnancy. Metronidazole may pass into breast milk and should therefore not be used during lactation.

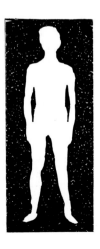

Always investigate
sexual contact

Since *T vaginalis* infestation is usually sexually acquired and often occurs concurrently with other sexually transmitted infections—for example, with gonorrhoea in 19% of cases—it should never be treated without full microbiological investigations and examination of regular sexual contacts. The organism is extremely difficult to identify in the male urethra, and usually the contacts are given a course of metronidazole even if trichomonads cannot be detected after examination and testing. This does not, however, imply that contacts should be treated by proxy. In view of the high incidence of associated infections all regular contacts should be seen and have microbiological tests performed.

Other infections

Management

Uncomplicated gonorrhoea
  Penicillin

Chlamydial infections
  Tetracycline

Contacts of men with chlamydia
    negative non-gonococcal urethritis
  Tetracycline

Anaerobic vaginosis
  Metronidazole

Both uncomplicated gonococcal and chlamydial infections in women are treated as for men (see previous chapter) with the same doses of penicillin or tetracycline. Female contacts of men with chlamydia negative non-gonococcal urethritis should be treated with tetracycline despite the absence of an organism.

Anaerobic vaginosis should be treated with metronidazole 400 mg twice daily for five days. Since the condition may be sexually acquired ideally male contacts should also be seen, particularly if the woman has recurrent attacks.

Management by the non-specialist

Epidemiological studies and ad hoc surveys of women attending gynaecology, obstetric, and family planning clinics indicate that candidiasis is more common than either trichomoniasis or gonorrhoea. Nevertheless, studies in departments of genitourinary medicine indicate that gonorrhoea, trichomoniasis, and candidiasis may occur concurrently. For these reasons the non-specialist may adopt various methods of management of genitourinary symptoms, depending on his own circumstances and the availability of laboratory facilities.

The academic approach—Because the common conditions causing vaginal discharge with or without vulval irritation may occur concurrently microbiological specimens should ideally be taken from all patients presenting with vaginal discharge. A speculum should be passed and endocervical and vaginal specimens obtained (see previous chapter). If the doctor has a microscope and Gram staining facilities he can exclude candidiasis, trichomoniasis, and gonorrhoea. Microscopy is fallible in all of these infections and specimens should be sent to the laboratory. Unless a microscopic diagnosis is made treatment should be withheld until the results have returned from the laboratory.

The realistic approach would be to perform the tests as above but to start treatment at the first consultation on the basis of the patient's history, absence or presence and type of symptoms in the sexual partner(s), examination, and the knowledge that common things occur commonly—namely candidiasis. This course should be followed only if the doctor insists on a follow up visit to assess the patient's progress and determine whether the correct treatment has been given in the light of the microbiological results.

For both the academic and realistic approaches contact tracing is an essential aspect of managing a sexually acquired infection. Both the source of infection and those who may in turn have been infected by the patient should be traced. The non-specialist often forgets that for each patient sitting in front of him there are at least two others infected in the community.

The pragmatic approach—Vaginal discharge with or without vulval irritation is a common presenting symptom and is most often due to an infection with *Candida albicans*. Therefore empirical treatment may be given without microbiological confirmation. This approach is contrary to that practised by the genitourinary physician, and, although the ideal would be to carry out microbiological investigations on all patients, limitation of resources and time may preclude this. This approach is reasonable so long as three fail safe mechanisms are observed. Firstly, an accurate clinical and sexual history must be taken to identify the high risk patient who needs tests or referral (see previous chapter). Secondly, treat for candidiasis alone so as not to mask other infections. The third failsafe mechanism is to insist that the patient returns for follow up after treatment. If symptoms are still present a concurrent sexually transmitted disease or wrong initial diagnosis may be a possibility, and the patient will need microbiological tests or referral to a department of genitourinary medicine.

The pragmatic approach is treatment before diagnosis and is acceptable only for low risk patients who will return for reassessment after treatment.

Vaginal discharge: management

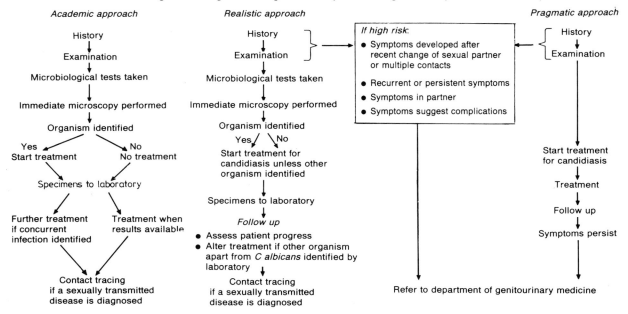

Management of vaginal discharge outside departments of genitourinary medicine

Academic approach

History
↓
Examination
↓
Microbiological tests taken
↓
Immediate microscopy performed
↓
Organism identified

Yes / No
Start treatment / No treatment
↓
Specimens to laboratory

Further treatment / Treatment when
if concurrent / results available
infection identified
↓
Contact tracing
if a sexually transmitted
disease is diagnosed

Realistic approach

History
↓
Examination
↓
Microbiological tests taken
↓
Immediate microscopy performed
↓
Organism identified

Yes / No
Start treatment for
candidiasis unless other
organism identified
↓
Specimens to laboratory
↓
Follow up
● Assess patient progress
● Alter treatment if other organism
apart from *C albicans* identified by
laboratory
↓
Contact tracing
if a sexually transmitted
disease is diagnosed

If high risk:
● Symptoms developed after
recent change of sexual partner
or multiple contacts
● Recurrent or persistent symptoms
● Symptoms in partner
● Symptoms suggest complications

↓
Refer to department of genitourinary medicine

Pragmatic approach

History
Examination
↓
Start treatment
for candidiasis
↓
Treatment
↓
Follow up
↓
Symptoms persist

COMPLICATIONS OF COMMON GENITAL INFECTIONS AND INFECTIONS IN OTHER SITES

Complications	Infection		
	Gonococcal	Chlamydia Positive	Negative
Women			
Local: Pelvic inflammatory disease	+	+	+
Bartholinitis/abscess	+	−	−
Systemic: Disseminated infection	+	−	−
Men			
Local: Epididymitis/orchitis	+	+	+
Prostatitis (± vesiculitis)	+	+	+
Systemic: Reiter's disease	−	+	+
Disseminated infection	+	−	−

If patients are treated early complications rarely occur. When they arise they are usually associated with chlamydia positive or chlamydia negative non-gonococcal infections or gonorrhoea and may be local or systemic.

Local complications: pelvic inflammatory disease

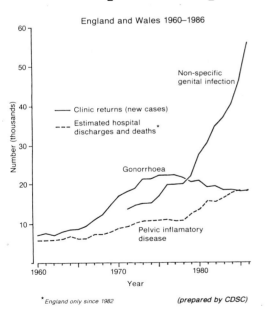

England and Wales 1960–1986

Number (thousands) / Year

— Clinic returns (new cases)
--- Estimated hospital discharges and deaths *

Non-specific genital infection

Gonorrhoea

Pelvic inflamatory disease

*England only since 1982

(prepared by CDSC)

Pelvic inflammatory disease

Symptoms:	Signs:
Lower abdominal pain	Fever
Malaise	Abdominal tenderness
Vaginal discharge	Adnexal tenderness ± pelvic mass
Dyspareunia, dysmenorrhoea	Cervical motion tenderness
	Purulent cervical discharge

Pelvic inflammatory disease is the most important complication associated with these three types of infection. About 10% of patients develop this complication after a gonococcal or non-gonococcal infection. In England and Wales the number of cases admitted to hospital has trebled in the past 25 years. In the United States the estimated direct costs of such hospital admissions alone are $900 m a year. In some African countries up to 45% of gynaecological admissions are due to this condition. In all of these countries many more cases are managed on an outpatient basis, for which no routine statistics are available.

Long term morbidity after recovery from acute pelvic inflammatory disease is considerable: chronic abdominal pain, menstrual disturbances, dyspareunia, infertility, tubal pregnancy, medical consultation and medication, time off work, and psychological sequelae. The most disastrous consequence of salpingitis is sterility. The proportion of patients with salpingitis who develop tubal occlusion rises from 10–13% with a first attack to 75% with three or more.

The diagnosis of pelvic inflammatory disease is often difficult. Clinically there is a combination of symptoms and signs, but even when these are correlated with laparoscopic findings the clinical diagnosis is correct in only 65% of patients. The condition is most often confused with appendicitis, endometriosis, and ectopic pregnancy.

Since acute pelvic inflammatory disease is often the direct result of a sexually transmitted infection, full microbiological tests must be carried out to detect infection with *Chlamydia trachomatis* or *Neisseria gonorrhoae*.

In all cases patients should be encouraged to rest in bed, even if they are not admitted to hospital. Any intrauterine device should be removed once treatment has started.

Complications and other infections

Non-gonococcal salpingitis:	tetracycline + metronidazole
Gonococcal infections:	benzylpenicillin, procaine penicillin, or ampicillin (if penicillin allergy–tetracycline, erythromycin, or co-trimoxazole)
Penicillinase producing *N gonorrhoeae:*	cefuroxime, or spectinomycin

Tetracycline is the drug of choice for either chlamydia positive or chlamydia negative non-gonococcal salpingitis (details are given in the box at the end of the chapter). Since these two types of infection are often polymicrobial, metronidazole should also be given to eradicate any possible anaerobic infection. If the patient has severe pelvic inflammatory disease—for example, pelvic peritonitis—it may be necessary to start treatment intravenously before using oral regimens.

Gonococcal infections need initial treatment with intramuscular benzylpenicillin or procaine penicillin or oral ampicillin and probenecid followed by ampicillin with probenecid. Alternatively, treatment with intramuscular penicillin may be continued until there are signs of clinical improvement (usually within 48 hours) before ampicillin is given. Finally, intravenous treatment may be indicated.

Gonococcal and chlamydial infections may occur together, and treatment with penicillin will only partially resolve the salpingitis. In such cases tetracycline should be given with metronidazole. The US Centers for Disease Control recommend that a broad spectrum combination of antibiotics should be used from the outset to eradicate *N gonorrhoeae* and *C trachomatis* with or without anaerobes. Thus examples of inpatient therapy would be intravenous doxycycline and cefoxitin or gentamicin and clindamycin and on an outpatient basis cefoxitin or ampicillin as an immediate dose followed by doxycycline or tetracycline by mouth for 10–14 days. This belt and braces approach is partly dictated by the fact that most patients with pelvic inflammatory disease in the USA are treated by private physicians, who often have no special knowledge of sexually acquired disease or access to microbiological support services.

For penicillinase producing strains of *N gonorrhoeae* cefuroxime or spectinomycin is the drug of choice. If a patient with gonococcal salpingitis is allergic to penicillin then tetracycline, erythromycin, or co-trimoxazole may be used.

All sexual contacts of the patient should be traced, to prevent infection of others and reinfection of the patient. Seeing contacts in this way and taking specimens for microbiological tests also help in identifying likely causative organisms which may have been missed in the female partner.

Local complications: vulva

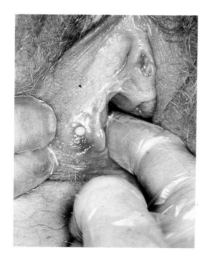

Bartholinitis or Bartholin's abscess is an uncommon complication of gonorrhoea. The patient may present with labial pain and swelling and sometimes difficulty in walking. Early in the condition pus may be visible or may be massaged out of the duct. Once an abscess has formed, however, a fluctuant mass will be felt. Specimens of pus should be collected from the duct (if draining), cervix, and urethra for microscopy and culture to isolate the gonococcus. *C trachomatis* should also be looked for since it may coexist with *N gonorrhoeae*. If *N gonorrhoeae* is identified and the duct is draining without an abscess having formed the patient should be treated with one intramuscular dose of either benzylpenicillin (5 MU) or procaine penicillin (2·4 MU), or oral ampicillin 2–3 g followed by ampicillin 500 mg four times a day for five to seven days. Probenicid should be given in association with penicillin. An abscess will not resolve adequately on antibiotics alone and marsupialisation is necessary to avoid further abscess formation. Sexual contacts should be investigated and urethral tests performed since, as with pelvic inflammatory disease, these often help in identifying the aetiological agent and preventing spread of the disease and reinfection.

Local complications: epididymis and testis

Differential diagnoses—epididymo-orchitis

Testicular torsion	Neoplasm
Urinary tract infection	Tubercle
Viral infection	

Epididymitis and orchitis due to a sexually transmitted agent are now rare. Patients with either condition or a combination (epididymo-orchitis) may also have a urethral discharge, but this is not invariable. A diagnosis of testicular torsion, urinary tract infection, neoplasm, or tubercle and viral infections affecting the testes (mumps, coxsackie, etc) should not be overlooked.

If gonorrhoea is confirmed by microscopy or culture of a sample of urethral discharge the usual treatment regimen of an initial dose of intramuscular or oral penicillin followed by oral ampicillin or probenecid for seven days should be given. Non-gonococcal infections should be treated with tetracycline 500 mg four times a day for two weeks. A scrotal support should be worn and in severe cases bed rest is necessary. Sexual contacts should be seen and investigated for chlamydia and gonorrhoea.

Local complications: prostate

Symptoms of prostatitis

Acute
  Pyrexia ± rigors
  Dysuria
  Frequency
  Urgency
  Perianal pain

Chronic
  Pain (suprapubic, perineal,
    low back, scrotal, thighs,
    penile tip, on ejaculation)
  Dysuria
  Frequency/nocturia
  Urgency
  Haematuria
  Haemospermia
  Low libido, impotence
  Depression

Minocycline   100 mg twice a day for 2 weeks

Doxycycline   100 mg a day for 2-3 weeks

Erythromycin 250 mg four times a day for 3-4 weeks

Tetracycline   250 mg four times a day for 3-4 weeks

Prostatitis may be associated with gonococcal and non-gonococcal infections as well as with a urinary tract infection. Chronic prostatitis is more common than acute prostatitis. Though rare, prostatitis associated with gonorrhoea is usually acute. In acute disease frequency of micturition, dysuria, urgency, and fever are more common symptoms than pain. On the other hand, in chronic prostatitis, which is usually caused by chlamydia positive or chlamydia negative non-gonococcal infections, pain is the most troublesome symptom; it may be suprapubic, perianal, lumbar, or scrotal; affect the thighs or tip of the penis; or be noticed only on ejaculation. Dysuria, frequency of micturition, haemospermia, low libido, impotence, or depression may also occur.

An accurate clinical history, thorough physical examination, and microbiological tests are all important in establishing a diagnosis. The prostate is only rarely tender and enlarged on rectal examination, and this is usually found in association with acute rather than chronic prostatitis. To obtain a specimen of prostatic secretion for microscopy and culture the prostate needs to be massaged. This procedure can precipitate an epididymitis in the presence of a posterior urethritis or cystitis and should not be carried out unless the second of the two glass urine test is clear.

The method used to obtain a specimen of prostatic fluid varies from straightforward massage to the Stamey technique of collecting urine both before and after the massage to differentiate between prostatitis, cystitis, and urethritis. More than 10 leucocytes per high power field ($\times 40$ magnification) or clumping of the cells, or both, in the prostatic secretion will indicate prostatitis. Further investigations of the urinary tract are indicated if a urinary tract infection is discovered.

If no organisms are identified on microscopy or culture of the prostatic fluid a broad spectrum antibiotic which is lipid soluble and so diffuses into the prostate should be given—for example, minocycline, doxycycline, or erthryomycin. Tetracycline may be given, but it is less effective as it does not penetrate the prostate well.

19

Complications and other infections

Systemic complications

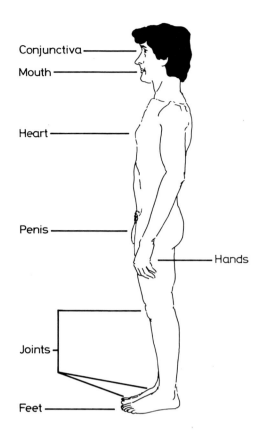

Disseminated gonococcal infection

Admit to hospital
Give high doses of penicillin
Trace all sexual contacts

Occasionally patients may present with or develop two rare but serious complications affecting multiple sites.

Reiter's disease

Reiter's disease, which is a seronegative polyarthropathy occurring as a rare (0·5–1%) complication of non-gonococcal urethritis, affects mainly men. *C trachomatis*, *Shigella*, *Salmonella*, and *Yersinia* have also been implicated in the aetiology of this condition. Conjunctivitis may also occur with the urethritis and arthritis but it is not an essential feature of the condition. The leg joints, particularly knees, ankles, and feet, are those most commonly affected. Other manifestations are mucous membrane lesions of the mouth and penis (circinate balanitis), keratodermia blenorrhagica of the feet and hands, onycholysis and ridging of the nails, and, rarely, pericarditis, partial heart block, aortic incompetence, peripheral neuropathy, and meningoencephalitis. An accurate clinical history is essential to exclude other arthropathies, such as rheumatoid arthritis and ankylosing spondylitis and those occurring with psoriasis, Crohn's disease, and ulcerative colitis.

Non-steroidal anti-inflammatory agents are given in mild cases—for example, indomethacin 25 mg three times a day. Bed rest, but not total immobilisation, is recommended during the active phase of the disease. Systemic steroids should be reserved for seriously ill patients or for those with complications such as pericarditis and uveitis. A concurrent non-gonococcal urethritis should be treated with tetracycline. The prognosis of Reiter's disease is extremely variable and relapses do occur.

Disseminated gonococcal infection

Disseminated gonococcal infection is a rare complication of gonorrhoea and affects women more often than men. The common symptoms are pain in the joints (wrists, knees, elbows, ankles, or small joints of the hand), tenosynovitis, and rash. The initial erythematous macular papular lesions develop into frank vesicles and pustules; they appear as crops on the trunk and arms and legs and often in association with a fever. Occasionally endocarditis, myocarditis, pericarditis, and meningitis may occur. Gonococci are often isolated from the genital tract and occasionally from blood and joint fluid but rarely from skin lesions. Patients need to be admitted to hospital and treated with high doses of penicillin. All sexual contacts must be traced.

Infections in other sites

Rectum—The rectum may be affected in several sexually transmitted conditions (gonorrhoea, chlamydia, non-gonococcal infection, genital herpes and warts, syphilis, *Entamoeba histolytica*, *Giardia lamblia*, and trauma). Only gonorrhoea is considered in this chapter. Rectal gonorrhoea is often symptomless and illustrates the need for contact tracing and regular check ups for homosexuals who are having casual sexual encounters. Symptoms, when they occur, are anal discomfort and pain, painful defecation, and a blood stained or purulent rectal discharge. Diagnosis is by microscopy and culture. Microscopy is incorrect in half of all cases since it is difficult to identify gonococci in the presence of many other organisms in the rectum. Cultures must always be performed if rectal gonorrhoea is suspected. Treatment and follow up of rectal gonorrhoea are the same as those for uncomplicated urethral or cervical infections.

Throat—Even though still uncommon, oropharyngeal gonorrhoea is being seen more often and may be asymptomatic. Patients admitting to orogenital contact will have throat swabs taken in a clinic in an attempt to isolate *N gonorrhoeae*. Patients with infection of the throat but no other site may also infect their partner's urethra during fellatio. Diagnosis is by culture; microscopy is useless owing to the presence of mixed organisms, particularly commensal neisseriae. In patients with pharyngeal infection high doses of penicillin or other antibiotics are needed to eradicate the organism. Ampicillin 3 g plus 1 g probenicid followed by 500 mg ampicillin four times a day for three days, co-trimoxazole (two tablets three times a day for seven days), or ciprofloxacin 250 mg immediately by mouth are recommended treatments.

Treatment of acute pelvic inflammatory disease

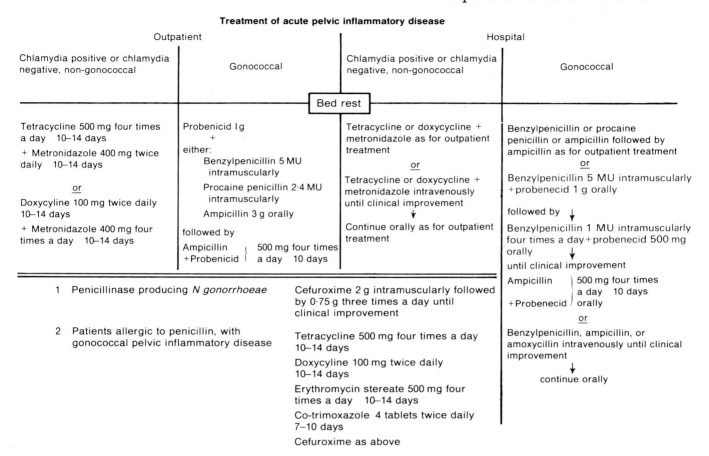

	Outpatient		Hospital	
	Chlamydia positive or chlamydia negative, non-gonococcal	Gonococcal	Chlamydia positive or chlamydia negative, non-gonococcal	Gonococcal

Bed rest

Outpatient — Chlamydia positive or chlamydia negative, non-gonococcal

Tetracycline 500 mg four times a day   10–14 days
+ Metronidazole 400 mg twice daily   10–14 days

or

Doxycyline 100 mg twice daily 10–14 days
+ Metronidazole 400 mg four times a day   10–14 days

Outpatient — Gonococcal

Probenicid I g
+
either:
  Benzylpenicillin 5 MU intramuscularly
  Procaine penicillin 2·4 MU intramuscularly
  Ampicillin 3 g orally
followed by
Ampicillin + Probenicid   500 mg four times a day   10 days

Hospital — Chlamydia positive or chlamydia negative, non-gonococcal

Tetracycline or doxycycline + metronidazole as for outpatient treatment

or

Tetracycline or doxycycline + metronidazole intravenously until clinical improvement
↓
Continue orally as for outpatient treatment

Hospital — Gonococcal

Benzylpenicillin or procaine penicillin or ampicillin followed by ampicillin as for outpatient treatment

or

Benzylpenicillin 5 MU intramuscularly + probenecid 1 g orally

followed by ↓

Benzylpenicillin 1 MU intramuscularly four times a day + probenecid 500 mg orally ↓
until clinical improvement

Ampicillin + Probenecid   500 mg four times a day   10 days orally

or

Benzylpenicillin, ampicillin, or amoxycillin intravenously until clinical improvement
↓
continue orally

---

1   Penicillinase producing *N gonorrhoeae*

Cefuroxime 2 g intramuscularly followed by 0·75 g three times a day until clinical improvement

2   Patients allergic to penicillin, with gonococcal pelvic inflammatory disease

Tetracycline 500 mg four times a day 10–14 days

Doxycyline 100 mg twice daily 10–14 days

Erythromycin stereate 500 mg four times a day   10–14 days

Co-trimoxazole 4 tablets twice daily 7–10 days

Cefuroxime as above

The illustration of Bartholin's abscess is reproduced, by permission, from King A, Nicol C, Rodin P. *Venereal Diseases*, published by Baillière Tindall.

GENITAL ULCERATION

Multiple and painful	Solitary and painful
Multiple and painless	Solitary and painless

Genital ulceration (or erosion) is a common symptom in both sexes and is often due to a sexually transmitted agent. Particular points that need to be elicited from the patient to aid diagnosis are the number of ulcers, the time they have been present, the degree of discomfort they cause and the relation of their appearance to sexual intercourse, trauma, and lesions elsewhere. Most ulcers or erosions are either multiple and painful or solitary and painless.

Multiple painful ulcers

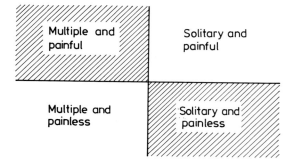
Primary herpes

Multiple ulcers, particularly if painful, are at present in the United Kingdom most commonly due to an infection with herpes simplex virus. If this is the patient's first attack the ulcers occur within one to two weeks of exposure to infection. The patient feels ill and the inguinal lymph nodes are enlarged, discrete, and usually painful. A recurrent attack is unlikely to bear any relation to sexual intercourse; it is sometimes preceded by prodromal symptoms and the patient often volunteers the diagnosis. Herpes zoster rarely gives rise to genital ulceration (see next chapter).

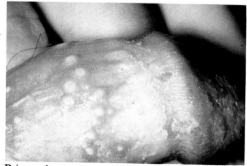
Behçet's disease

Other causes of painful multiple ulcers are Behçet's disease and, rarely in the United Kingdom, chancroid caused by *Haemophilus ducreyi*. Behçet's disease is usually associated with oral ulcers and chancroid is invariably contracted abroad or from a sexual partner who has recently returned from abroad. Chancroid has an extremely short incubation period of two to five days. Scabies may also rarely present as multiple, itching, painful, secondarily infected ulcerated papules produced by scratching.

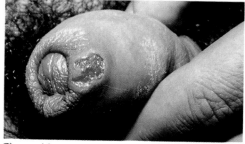
Chancroid

Patients with non-gonococcal, gonococcal, trichomonal, and candidal infections may have multiple painful erosive lesions on the penis and vulva, sometimes with fissuring. Balanitis and vulvitis may also be found in infections with β haemolytic streptococci and Vincent's organisms. Similar lesions may occur as part of the Stevens–Johnson or Reiter's syndrome, or be due to erythema multiforme, dermatitis, psoriasis and lichen planus, impetigo, furuncles, folliculitis, and drug eruptions.

Solitary painless ulcers

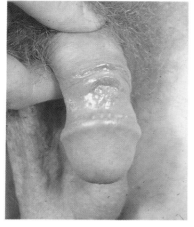

Primary syphilis

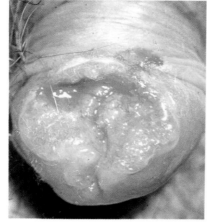

Carcinoma of penis

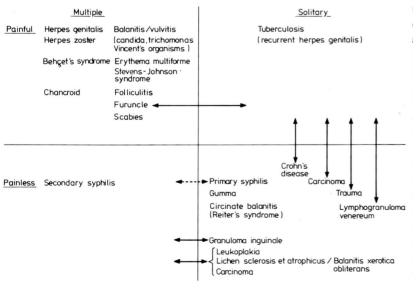

Lymphogranuloma venereum

The commonest cause of painless genital ulceration is primary syphilis. The incubation period is usually 21 days but the lesions may appear from nine to 90 days after sexual intercourse with an infected partner. Inguinal lymph nodes are moderately enlarged, painless, and discrete. Other stages of syphilis may also result in genital ulceration. Ulcers of the secondary stage, evident as eroded papules or mucous patches, will be multiple but painless, whereas a gumma is usually solitary, painless, and a tertiary manifestation. Other causes of solitary painless ulcers are carcinoma, circinate balanitis, balanitis xerotica obliterans, lymphogranuloma venereum, and granuloma inguinale. Self inflicted trauma or dermatitis artefacta may give rise to large solitary ulcerated areas which are surprisingly painless. More traumatic lesions of the penis, anus, and rectum usually result from sadomasochistic practices.

Diagnosis

The two commonest causes of genital ulceration in the United Kingdom are herpes and syphilis. These often look different on macroscopic examination, but the naked eye should not be relied on to differentiate between them or confirm the diagnosis. Herpes is diagnosed by culture of the virus. To exclude primary or secondary syphilis three separate specimens of serum from the ulcer(s) should be examined by dark ground microscopy initially and on three consecutive days. Serological tests for syphilis are not always positive when primary syphilitic lesions are present; the tests do not become positive for about three to four weeks after infection, whereas a primary lesion or chancre may be evident as soon as nine to ten days after exposure.

If the ulceration is due to circinate balanitis, scabies, or Behçet's syndrome, other extragenital lesions may usually be found. The three tropical conditions of chancroid, lymphogranuloma venereum, and granuloma inguinale require special culture facilities. In addition to investigating the cause of the presenting symptom of genital ulceration, tests must be carried out to exclude other concurrent sexually transmitted diseases contracted at the same time and to determine the underlying cause of the ulcers or erosions.

Causes of genital ulceration and erosions

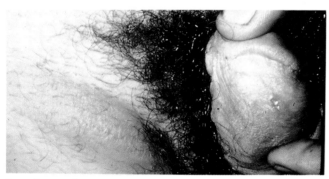

	Multiple		Solitary
Painful	Herpes genitalis	Balanitis/vulvitis (candida, trichomonas Vincent's organisms)	Tuberculosis (recurrent herpes genitalis)
	Herpes zoster		
	Behçet's syndrome	Erythema multiforme Stevens-Johnson syndrome	
	Chancroid	Folliculitis	
		Furuncle	
		Scabies	
Painless	Secondary syphilis	Primary syphilis Gumma Circinate balanitis (Reiter's syndrome)	Crohn's disease Carcinoma Trauma Lymphogranuloma venereum
		Granuloma inguinale Leukoplakia Lichen sclerosis et atrophicus / Balanitis xerotica obliterans Carcinoma	

GENITAL HERPES

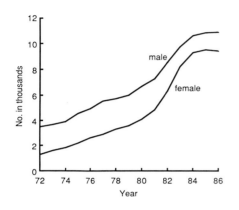

The problems associated with genital herpes

Increasing

No curative treatment

Recurrent

Breakdown of relationships/psychosexual
problems/depression

Neonatal infections

Genital infection with herpes simplex virus poses five problems. It is increasing, it is an unpleasant disease with no cure, and it is recurrent, the last two of which may lead to breakdown of relationships, psychosexual problems, and depression; and, finally, it may cause neonatal and possibly fetal infections.

The latest figures (1987) show that 17 966 cases of genital herpes were seen in departments of genitourinary medicine in the United Kingdom. The number of cases has levelled off in recent years. These figures make it the fourth most common sexually transmitted disease. Certainly, more cases exist than are diagnosed in departments of genitourinary medicine and these will be managed in general practice or by gynaecologists and dermatologists. In the United States of America no uniform or universal data are collected. However, it is estimated that there are between 200 000 and 500 000 new cases of herpes each year and a total of about 40 million sufferers in all.

The virus

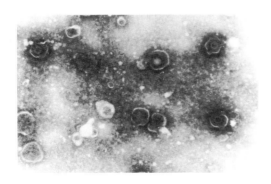

Herpes simplex virus is a double stranded DNA virus which can be classified into types 1 and 2. Both types can cause genital infection even though type 1 usually causes lesions of the face, lips, and eyes. The prevalence of type 1 infection varies inversely with socioeconomic state. Type 1 and type 2 antibodies are thought to offer some cross protection, and the reduction in type 1 infection and antibody development during childhood in developed countries may be a factor in the increase in genital herpes in such countries.

The virus is transmitted by sexual intercourse or other physical contact. Orogenital contact with a partner with type 1 labial lesions may result in genital herpes. The illness may range from being entirely asymptomatic to being a severe systemic and mucocutaneous disease.

Primary infections

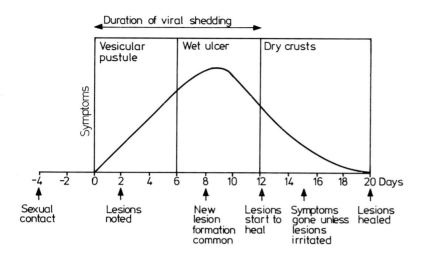

A first attack (primary herpes) of genital herpes usually presents with multiple painful genital ulcers after a short incubation period of under seven days. The amount of pain experienced by the patient varies depending on the number and site of the lesions. All the skin lesions, whether on the genitals themselves or on adjacent areas (buttocks, thighs, anus), evolve in the same way—starting with erythema, progressing to vesicles then ulcers, and finishing with crusting. The separate lesions often coalesce into substantial areas of shallow ulceration. These local lesions and viral shedding last about 12 days, with healing taking a further week, so that the whole illness may last for three weeks. In most primary attacks in women both the vulva and the cervix are affected (80–90% of cases). Nevertheless, single sites may be affected so that cervical lesions may be present without vulval lesions and vice versa.

Inguinal lymphadenopathy occurs in most primary cases and about half of these patients actually complain of pain in the groin. Anorectal herpes can cause pain, discharge, and constipation. About one third of patients may have vague constitutional symptoms of fever and malaise and about 10% headache, photophobia, and viral meningitis. Retention of urine is a very rare symptom and in most instances is due to the patient's understandable reluctance to pass urine over already painful lesions; occasionally it is due to the virus affecting the sacral autonomic plexus, with a resulting meningomyelitis.

Site	Symptoms					
	Pain	Dysuria	Retention	Constipation	Discharge	None
Penis (glans, coronal sulcus and shaft)	+					±
Urethra (male)	++	+	+		+	+
Anus/rectum	+		±	+	+	+
Buttocks/thighs/scrotum	+					
Vulva/urethra	++	+	±		±	±
Vagina	+				+	±
Cervix	+				++	+

Recurrent infections

Recurrent infections are less severe and are not due to reinfection. Patients offer a variety of precipitating causes for their recurrences such as stress, sexual intercourse, menstruation, and climatic changes. Epidemiological data suggest that the mean time interval between initial and recurrent infection is about 120 days (range 25–360 days). The rate of recurrence, however, is to some extent dependent on viral type. Patients with HSV 2 tend to suffer recurrences earlier after the primary infection and then more frequently than those with type 1 infection. Patients often notice prodromal symptoms of local tingling and parasthesiae for 24–48 hours before the onset of lesions. The recurrent infection is not only milder but also shorter than the initial attack. There are fewer, but identical, lesions which heal more rapidly than previously. Systemic manifestations are rare.

Patients with both initial and recurrent attacks may be asymptomatic, unaware that they have infection or have minor complaints which are not attributed to herpes. Some studies suggest that up to 50% of patients fall into these groups. This raises considerable problems not only for the patient but also in relation to control of the disease within the community.

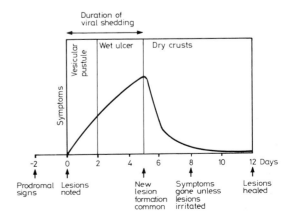

Genital herpes

The diagnosis

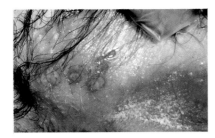

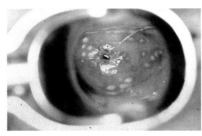

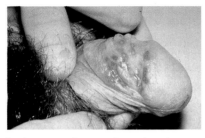

Lesions on vulva, cervix, and penis

The clinical history and examination usually give the doctor a good idea of the eventual diagnosis. Nevertheless, the ulceration has to be differentiated from syphilis by dark ground microscopy. Other sexually transmitted diseases such as gonorrhoea, chlamydial infections, and trichomoniasis, which could have been contracted at the same time, must be excluded by full microbiological tests. Serological tests for syphilis should be taken as a base line, as should cervical cytology.

Even though women may complain only of vulval lesions, the cervix must be visualised since it is affected in 80–90% of cases of primary disease. The cervix may be ulcerated, frankly necrotic, or appear normal, and since in all instances the virus can be grown specimens should be taken from both the vulva and cervix in all patients. The definitive diagnosis of genital herpes can be made only by viral culture and isolation of the organism. Newer immunoassays are becoming increasingly available for diagnosis. They are not so sensitive as culture but have the advantage of speed and the ability to type the virus. Similarly, a homosexual patient who complains only of anal lesions should be examined with a proctoscope to ascertain the extent of the disease and have tests carried out for herpes and other sexually transmitted conditions.

Material for culture should be taken with a sterile cotton wool swab which is rubbed over the lesions so that adequate serum is obtained. If only vesicles are present, one or two of them may need to be punctured to obtain the specimen. This should be placed in a viral transport medium, refrigerated at 4°C, and sent to the laboratory on the same day. Since herpes is a chronic and incurable infection the diagnosis must always be confirmed by culture. It is unfair to the patient as well as to his or her sexual contacts to make such a diagnosis purely on clinical grounds. These may mislead, and a wrong diagnosis may create unnecessary anxiety for more than one person.

Routine management

Bathe lesions in warm saline

Analgesics

Treat secondary infections

Admit to hospital if:

Uncontrollable pain

Urinary retention

? Meningitis

The treatment of genital herpes still remains unsatisfactory and no cure is yet available. The conservative palliative approach should be the basis of management. To some extent pain may be alleviated by bathing the lesions in warm saline (a teaspoon of domestic salt added to 0·5 l of warm tap water); this also helps to keep the lesions clean. If the lesions are particularly severe patients may be encouraged to sit in a warm bath to which salt has been added (three tablespoons). Patients often find that swishing the water around the lesions while sitting in the bath is soothing and that it is easier to pass urine. Pain may also be relieved by simple analgesics, and some patients find relief by the use of ice packs. Occasionally secondary infection occurs and should be treated with an appropriate antibiotic such as co-trimoxazole. This antibiotic has the advantage of being non-treponemicidal and will, therefore, not mask syphilis. Some patients are so ill, usually during the initial attack, that they require admission to hospital. The indications for this are uncontrollable pain, urinary retention, and possible meningitis.

Antiviral agents and vaccines

Treatment

Ineffective – idoxuridine

Possibly prove effective – acylovir, vaccines

Do not use steroids

Several agents have been introduced over recent years with claims that they are antiviral and change the disease process. The best known of these is idoxuridine, which is expensive and of no use in genital, as opposed to labial, herpes. Recently an antiviral agent, acyclovir, has been introduced which acts on a specific viral enzyme thus preventing viral replication. Studies using this drug in primary and recurrent attacks have shown that viral shedding, healing time, and duration of symptoms may be reduced but that the subsequent development of recurrences is not affected. At present oral acyclovir is useful in primary attacks. Recurrences can only be prevented by continuous prophylactic use. This is expensive and not advisable until data on long term safety are available. No effective vaccine presently exists; those being developed still need to be tested by randomised controlled trials.

Counselling and other problems

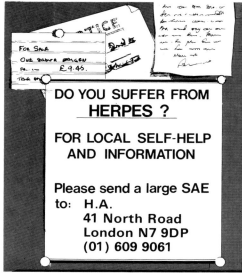

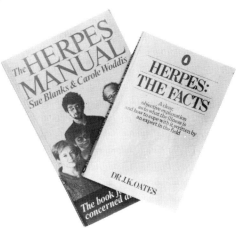

Genital herpes is an emotive disease, particularly since it is recurrent and may interfere with sexual intercourse. Patients often need a great deal of advice and emotional support and since the condition is incurable, it is important that dotors at least fulfil these two functions. Patients should be warned that they are infectious when lesions are present; they should therefore abstain from sexual intercourse once lesions are noted or sooner if prodromal symptoms are present. Since lesions are widespread, particularly in women, the sheath will not always stop contact with infected areas and is not therefore effective in preventing infection during an attack. Since asymptomatic infection and viral shedding can exist the regular use of condoms between overt attacks will need to be discussed with patients. Likewise patients should be reminded that other forms of intimacy and close bodily contact, apart from sexual intercourse, are not precluded. They often find it useful to talk to fellow sufferers, and the recent creation of the Herpes Association, acting as a self help counselling and information centre, is welcomed.

Two major concerns relating to genital herpes are the possible effects on the fetus and neonate and, in the long term, on the cervix. (The problems of in utero and neonatal infection are covered in a later chapter.)

The possibility of an association between herpes simplex virus type 2 infections and cervical neoplasms has been the subject of controversy for nearly two decades, and the relation is not fully established or proved. As long as doubt exists caution is recommended. Patients who have had genital herpes should have cytology performed initially and then at yearly intervals. This approach has to be weighed against the possibility of patients becoming neurotic about cancer. This may be avoided by explaining the current evidence and that any changes found by yearly cytology would be early ones, which are highly amenable to cure.

The illustrations of the clinical course of primary and recurrent infections were reproduced by permission of Dr L Corey.

VIRAL HEPATITIS

IAN WELLER

Causes

Hepatitis A	4–6 weeks' incubation
	Faecal-oral, sexual (homosexual) transmission
Hepatitis B	12 weeks' incubation
	Parenteral or percutaneous, perinatal, sexual (homosexual and heterosexual) transmission
	Carrier state
Non-A non-B	(a) 5 weeks' incubation
	Faecal-oral (epidemic) transmission
	(b) 8 weeks' incubation
	Parenteral or percutaneous transmission (?sexual)
	Carrier state

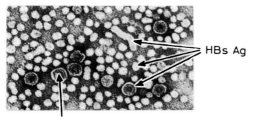

HBs Ag

HBc— contains DNA, DNA polymerase and e antigen (also free in serum)

Hepatitis B—groups at risk

- Endemic areas—whole population at early age
- Neonates of carrier mothers
- Homosexual men
- Prostitutes
- Intravenous drug abusers
- Sexual contact(s) of carriers
- Certain patients, laboratory and medical staff exposed to blood or blood products or in closed institutions

The four main viral causes of heptatitis are hepatitis A, hepatitis B, non-A non-B virus(es), and hepatitis D (previously delta agent). Cytomegalovirus and Epstein-Barr virus occasionally cause hepatitis.

Hepatitis A is caused by a small RNA virus, which is excreted in the stools for up to two weeks before the onset of symptoms. With increasing standards of hygiene in the developed world an older section of the population becomes susceptible. Fewer than a fifth of young heterosexual adults in London are immune. As a sexually transmitted infection hepatitis A occurs mainly among homosexual men because of oral-anal contact. Recovery is the rule after hepatitis A.

Hepatitis B virus is a DNA virus. It is usually present in serum many weeks before the acute illness. In populations with a high carrier rate—for example, tropical Africa and South East Asia, where 8–20% of people carry the virus—the whole population is at risk of infection. Much infection occurs perinatally or during early childhood. In populations with a low carrier rate, such as the United Kingdom, where about 1 in 1000 of the population carry the virus, only certain groups are at high risk of infection. As a sexually transmitted disease hepatitis B in the United Kingdom occurs largely in homosexual men. Risk factors are multiple casual sexual partners, anal intercourse, and a high carrier rate (about 5% in those attending departments of genitourinary medicine).

Hepatitis D virus is a defective RNA virus which needs hepatitis B virus to produce infection. Transmitted with hepatitis B it may be part of a dual acute infection, but more importantly it can occur as a superinfection in carriers of the B virus and may cause transient, severe acute, or fulminant hepatitis, or (in up to 90% of cases) chronic superinfection and worsened chronic liver disease. Although hepatitis D is thought to be more common in intravenous drug users and haemophiliacs, serological evidence of it has recently been reported in up to 14% of homosexual carriers of hepatitis B virus.

Non-A non-B virus(es) emerged as important causes of hepatitis once serological tests were available to identify A and B viruses, cytomegalovirus, and Epstein-Barr virus. There may be two agents transmitted via percutaneous routes, blood, and blood products. In developed countries the groups at risk are similar to those at risk of hepatitis B. A carrier state exists and is more common. Non-A non-B viruses account for 15–30% of cases of sporadic acute hepatitis. In 25–30% of patients there is no history of parenteral exposure and limited observations suggest occasional transmission by person to person and sexual contact. In homosexual men, however, the risks of hepatitis A and B are much higher. Chronicity after sporadic non-A non-B virus infection is unusual. A non-A non-B hepatitis spread by the oral-faecal route (enteric NANB) has caused waterborne epidemics in South East and central Asia, Africa, and North America. It has an incubation period similar to that of hepatitis A and no carrier state. Immune electron microscopy has shown 27–30 nm virus like particles in stools.

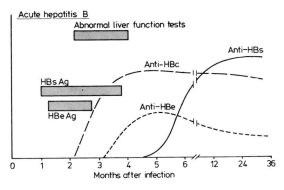

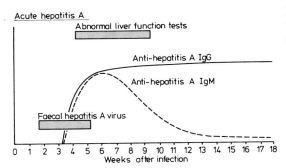

History and examination—It is important to inquire about sexual orientation and contacts and whether the partner has symptoms of hepatitis. Most cases of acute hepatitis diagnosed in departments of genitourinary medicine occur in homosexual men and are due to A or B viruses. A history of travel, intravenous drug abuse, tattoos, recent transfusion, or percutaneous exposure may also be relevant. Hepatotoxins such as alcohol and drugs should also be excluded as a cause of hepatitis. There are no major differences in the clinical features of acute hepatitis due to A, B, or non-A non-B viruses. More than half of acute infections are subclinical. The clinical illness begins with non-specific symptoms such as fever, headache, and fatigue, and jaundice follows. Symptoms and signs of other concurrent sexually transmitted diseases should be looked for.

Laboratory tests—Routine liver function tests are unhelpful in identifying the responsible virus; they may help to distinguish between hepatitis and cholestasis due to extrahepatic or intrahepatic lesions, but prolonged cholestasis does occur with viral hepatitis. Tests of synthetic function such as prothrombin time and serum albumin are useful in assessing the severity of the hepatitis.

Specific serological tests—Hepatitis A, Epstein-Barr virus, and cytomegalovirus infections are best diagnosed by tests for specific serum IgM antibodies, which persist for a short time and indicate recent infection. IgG antibodies appear more slowly, persist for many years, and indicate immunity. Early in acute hepatitis B, hepatitis B surface (HBsAg) and hepatitis B e antigens (HBeAg) appear in the serum. In a minority HBsAg may disappear before the onset of clinical symptoms. Anti-HBc appears during the acute illness followed by anti-HBe. Neither of these antibodies provide immunity. Anti-HBs, which provides long term immunity, appears after HBsAg has disappeared, though there may be a long gap. In this serological gap anti-HBc will be the only evidence of hepatitis B infection and IgM anti-HBc evidence of recent infection. In a patient with acute hepatitis detection of HBsAg will usually indicate acute B virus infection but in a few cases may represent some other cause of hepatitis in a B virus carrier. Until recently there were no specific serological tests for non-A non-B viruses and the diagnosis was one of exclusion. A serological test has been developed to show antibodies to the parenterally transmitted agent, which appears to be a single stranded RNA virus with a lipid envelope. The antibody test utilises a recombinant antigen from a DNA library obtained from a concentrated viral preparation of chimpanzee plasma. The assay seems to detect about 70% of cases of hepatitis acquired after transfusion. More sensitive and less cumbersome serological tests for antibodies to the enteric NANB virus are being developed.

Serological diagnosis of acute non-A non-B hepatitis	
Exclude alcohol and drugs etc	
HBsAg	negative
IgM antibodies to HBc	negative
IgM antibodies to HAV	negative
IgM antibodies to EBV	negative
IgM antibodies to CMV	negative

In all patients with hepatitis that may have been acquired sexually, other sexually transmitted diseases should be excluded by taking appropriate specimens for microscopy and culture from exposed sites and performing serological tests for syphilis.

Viral hepatitis

Complications

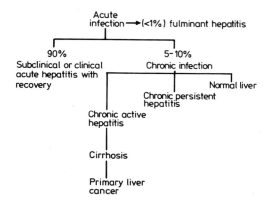

Fulminant hepatitis is a rare complication occurring in less than 1% of patients with acute viral hepatitis. Some 5–10% of patients with acute hepatitis B develop a chronic infection (HBsAg persists in serum for more than six months). Early in the chronic carrier state the complete virion, and therefore HBsAg and HBeAg, are present in the serum. These carriers are of high infectivity (supercarriers). Liver biopsy is the most reliable way of assessing whether the chronic carrier has a normal liver, chronic persistent hepatitis, chronic active hepatitis, or cirrhosis.

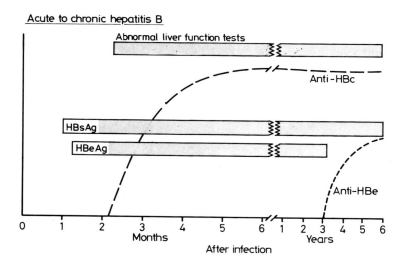

Chronic persistent hepatitis is usually benign. Some patients do, however, progress to chronic active hepatitis and cirrhosis, particularly if HBeAg remains in their serum. Longstanding chronic hepatitis B infection and the development of cirrhosis are associated with a high risk of primary hepatocellular carcinoma.

Management

Indications for admission to hospital
Complications
Symptoms and signs of acute liver
failure (earliest = neuropsychiatric)
Doubts about diagnosis
? extrahepatic cause for jaundice
Social factors
young adult living alone

Acute viral hepatitis is usually self limiting and management largely supportive. Most patients can be managed as outpatients, but acute liver failure and its complications demand urgent admission to intensive care.

In uncomplicated cases a low fat, high energy diet is more palatable and bed rest advisable during the early phase of the illness. Alcohol is excluded at least until liver function tests are normal.

In chronic hepatitis management is also largely supportive and antiviral treatment still experimental. Results of treatment with alfa interferon, however, are promising in patients with chronic hepatitis B, and responses are also being seen in those with chronic NANB and hepatitis D. Carriers with anti-HBe and normal biochemical and histological findings should be reassured. Alcohol even in moderation may hasten the progression of chronic liver disease.

Prevention

Because of the lack of specific treatment, prevention has been the main aim in managing viral hepatitis, especially hepatitis B. Simple hygienic precautions, in the case of hepatitis A, and careful handling of blood, blood contaminated material, and instruments, in the case of hepatitis B, will appreciably decrease transmission from patients.

Regular sexual contacts of patients with acute hepatitis A or B should be traced and offered passive immunisation. Ideally all those who have had sexual contact with a patient with acute hepatitis B in the preceding three months should be traced. Unidentified HBeAg positive carriers may then be found as a source of infection. These patients should be counselled about their infectivity and reduction in number of casual partners, and their non-immune regular sexual contacts should be vaccinated.

Hepatitis B vaccine—Purified, inactivated, alum conjugated 22 nm HBsAg particle and recombinant yeast vaccines are now available for high risk groups. They are safe and protect over 90% of young immunocompetent vaccinees for at least several years. The groups at risk are priority groups for vaccination. Savings can be made by pretesting for antibodies to HBs in those with high attack rates and pre-existing immunity, such as homosexuals, and by not doing so in those with low attack rates, such as certain medical staff.

Prevention of hepatitis as a sexually transmitted disease

Contact tracing
Counselling of HBeAg positive carriers

| Passive immunisation | Hepatitis A—normal pooled immunoglobulin |
| | Hepatitis B—hepatitis B immunoglobulin (HBIg) |

Active immunisation—vaccine

Interactions between infection with human immunodeficiency virus (HIV) and hepatitis B virus (HBV)

↓ HBV attack rate because of changing sexual behaviour

Interactions resulting from immunosuppression

? ↓ incidence of fulminant hepatitis

↑ infectivity of HBV carriers

↓ hepatic inflammatory activity

↓ response rate to vaccine

↑ loss of natural and vaccine induced antibodies

? ↓ response to antiviral treatment

? effect on risk of cirrhosis and hepatocellular carcinoma

Concomitant infections with hepatitis B and human immunodeficiency viruses are common. Documented and potential interactions between these two infections may therefore in future affect the epidemiology and natural history of HBV infection.

AIDS

IAN WELLER

Definition

Diseases diagnostic of AIDS if laboratory evidence of HIV exists
Diseases diagnosed definitively
Recurrent/multiple bacterial infections—child aged under 13
Coccidioidomycosis—disseminated
HIV encephalopathy
Histoplasmosis—disseminated
Isosporiasis—diarrhoea persisting > 1 month
Kaposi's sarcoma at any age
Primary cerebral lymphoma at any age
Non-Hodgkin's lymphoma—diffuse, undifferentiated B cell type, or unknown phenotype
Any disseminated mycobacterial disease caused by other than *M tuberculosis*
Mycobacterial tuberculosis—extrapulmonary
Salmonella septicaemia—recurrent
HIV wasting syndrome
Diseases diagnosed presumptively
Candidiasis—oesophageal
Cytomegalovirus retinitis with visual loss
Kaposi's sarcoma
Lymphoid interstitial pneumonia—child aged under 13
Mycobacterial disease (acid fast bacilli; species not identified by culture)—disseminated
Pneumocystis carinii pneumonia
Cerebral toxoplasmosis

AIDS is defined as an illness characterised by one or more indicator diseases. In the absence of another cause of immune deficiency and without laboratory evidence of HIV infection (if the patient has not been tested or the results are inconclusive), certain diseases when definitely diagnosed are indicative of AIDS. Regardless of the presence of other causes of immune deficiency, if there is laboratory evidence of HIV infection other indicator diseases that require a definitive, or in some cases only a presumptive, diagnosis also constitute a diagnosis of AIDS. The causative agent of AIDS is the human immunodeficiency virus (HIV).

Diseases diagnostic of AIDS without laboratory evidence of HIV
Candidiasis—oesophageal, pulmonary
Cryptococcosis—extrapulmonary
Cytomegalovirus disease—disseminated
Cryptosporidiosis—diarrhoea persisting > 1 month
Herpes simplex virus (HSV) infection
—mucocutaneous ulceration lasting > 1 month
—pulmonary, oesophageal infection
Kaposi's sarcoma—patient aged < 60
Primary cerebral lymphoma—patient aged < 60
Lymphoid interstitial pneumonia—child aged < 13
Mycobacterium avium ⎫ disseminated
Mycobacterium kansasii ⎭
Pneumocystis carinii pneumonia
Progressive multifocal leucoencephalopathy
Cerebral toxoplasmosis

Epidemiology

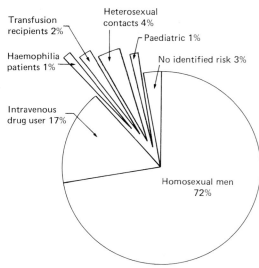

Groups affected in the USA

HIV is transmitted sexually, in blood or blood products, and perinatally. The number of reported cases continues to increase. By July/August 1989, 102 621 cases had been reported in the USA and 2561 in the UK. Most (94%) of those affected are men. Most of the affected women are intravenous drug abusers, have had sexual contact with intravenous drug abusers or bisexual men, or are from countries where heterosexual transmission is a prominent risk factor. Paediatric cases usually occur as a result of the mother having AIDS or belonging to a group at risk of AIDS, usually (76%) an intravenous drug user. The "no identified risk" group includes people for whom information is incomplete, for example, because of death or inadequate history.

In Europe a further risk group was identified when AIDS was reported in patients from central Africa. This reflected the appearance of the syndrome there, which has currently reached epidemic proportions although there is considerable under reporting of cases. Heterosexual intercourse is the main route of transmission with a ratio of men:women of virtually 1:1.

Immunology

Range of immune dysfunction

Lymphopenia ↓T helper (T4+/CD4+)
↓ Skin anergy to common recall antigens, such as Candida, PPD, tetanus
↓ Proliferative responses (mitogens, antigens, alloantigens)
↓ Cytotoxic responses—cell mediated T cell (T8)
                                natural killer cell
↓ Monocyte function
↑ Immunoglobulins—polyclonal B cell activation
                    ↓ de novo antibody response
↑ Circulating immune complexes

Others   autoantibodies
         ↑ acid labile interferon
         ↑ β2 microglobulin
         ↑ α₁ thymosin

A depletion or impaired function of the T helper or inducer lymphocyte subset (lymphocytes bearing the T4 or CD4 cluster differentiation antigen) seems to be the primary abnormality of immune dysfunction. The CD4 molecule, however, is also displayed at lower density on other cells such as monocytes, macrophages, and some B lymphocytes. The CD4 lymphocyte has a pivotal role in the immune response (interacting with macrophages, other T cells, B cells, and natural killer cells either by direct contact or via the influence of lymphokines such as gamma interferon and interleukin 2). The other immunological abnormalities seem to be largely secondary to the disorder of CD4 lymphocytes.

The virus

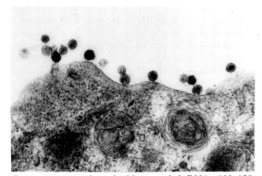

HIV has a cylindrical core. Its nucleic acid has been cloned and sequenced. It has a basic gene structure common to retroviruses but is very different from the other human retroviruses, human T lymphotropic viruses I and II. The CD4 antigen is a major component of the viral receptor required for cell entry. Only cells bearing this antigen are susceptible to infection. On entry to the infected cell the viral reverse transcriptase enzyme (hence retrovirus) makes a DNA copy (proviral DNA) of the RNA genome. The proviral DNA is able to integrate into the host cell DNA. Latent or non-productive or productive viral replication may occur. During productive replication RNA transcripts are made from the proviral DNA, and complete virus particles are assembled and released from infected cells by characeristic budding.

Properties: retrovirus double stranded RNA, 100–120 nm diameter; genes are *gag* (core proteins), *pol* (polymerase/reverse transcriptase), *env* (envelope proteins), and genes that regulate viral protein synthesis and replication; wide genomic diversity, most pronounced in *env* region. CD4 tropism; cytopathic effect in susceptible cell lines; latency; antibodies to core and envelope proteins (weak neutralising activity).

In vitro, HIV produces a cytopathic effect in susceptible cell lines, multinucleate giant cells (syncytia) form, and cell death occurs. The mechanism(s) by which it produces immune dysfunction in vivo are not yet clear.

Serological profile

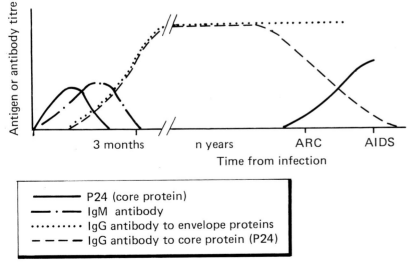

Time from infection (x-axis); *Antigen or antibody titre* (y-axis); 3 months, n years, ARC, AIDS

———— P24 (core protein)
—·—·— IgM antibody
············ IgG antibody to envelope proteins
— — — IgG antibody to core protein (P24)

Serological profile of infection with HIV

Acute viraema, detected by the presence of the core protein (P24), precedes the appearance of antibodies (IgG and IgM) to the "whole" virus. While the patient remains asymptomatic, high titres of antibodies to envelope and core proteins persist and P24 remains detectable in only about 10% of patients. As immune deficiency develops the titre of antibody to P24 falls but the titres of antibodies to the viral envelope proteins (GP 41, 120, and 160) remain high. P24 antigenaemia recurs with time and is found in 50–60% of patients with symptomatic disease.

AIDS

Natural history

Acute infection with HIV may be accompanied by a transient non-specific illness similar to glandular fever; it includes fever, malaise, myalgia, lymphadenopathy, pharyngitis, and a rash. A transient aseptic meningoencephalitis may also occur. Most acute infections, however, are subclinical. The acute infection is accompanied by the development of antibodies to the core and surface proteins, usually in two to six weeks, though delayed seroconversions have been observed. Antibodies are usually detected by enzyme linked immunoassays, and their presence can be confirmed by immunofluorescence or western blot.

A chronic infection ensues. This is asymptomatic in the early stages. Physical examination may show no abnormality, but about one third of patients have persistent generalised lymphadenopathy (nodes of 1 cm or more in diameter in two or more non-contiguous extrainguinal sites, which cannot be explained by any other infection or condition). The commonest sites of lymphadenopathy are the cervical and axillary lymph nodes; it is unusual in the hilar lymph nodes. Biopsy usually shows a benign profuse follicular hyperplasia.

Later in infection non-specific constitutional symptoms develop, which may be intermittent or persistent; they include fevers, night sweats, diarrhoea, and weight loss. Patients may also be affected by several "minor" opportunistic infections or conditions that tend to affect the mucous membranes and skin, such as oral candidiasis, oral hairy leucoplakia, herpes zoster, recurrent oral or anogenital herpes simplex, and other skin conditions such as seborrhoeic dermatitis, folliculitis, impetigo, and tinea infections. This collection of symptoms and signs, which are often a prodrome to the development of major opportunistic infection or tumour, are often referred to as AIDS related complex (ARC).

Prospective cohort studies have shown that several clinical and laboratory abnormalities carry a significant predictive value for the later development of AIDS. About 75% of HIV infected people can be expected to develop symptomatic (CDC group IV) disease in nine to 10 years.

Tumours

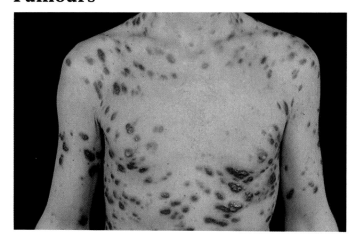

Kaposi's sarcoma

Kaposi's sarcoma is a presenting feature in 25% of patients, and is commoner in homosexual men than in the other groups at risk. The median survival time is about two years, though death is usually caused by a supervening life threatening opportunistic infection.

The Kaposi's sarcoma of AIDS differs from classic Kaposi's sarcoma in that widespread skin, mucous membrane (particularly the oral cavity and palate), visceral, and lymph node disease occurs. Visceral, particularly gastrointestinal, lesions are present in as many as half of all patients at presentation.

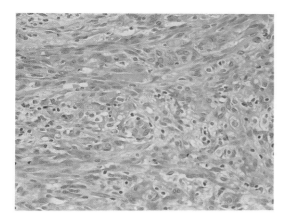

Spindle cell proliferation of nodular Kaposi's sarcoma

Nodules of Kaposi's sarcoma also occur in the lungs. Chest x ray appearances vary from confluent irregular masses to interstitial nodularity. Computed tomography of the thorax may be useful in differential diagnosis. At bronchoscopy, endobronchial lesions may be seen.

Kaposi's sarcoma consists of spindle shaped cells arranged in nodules and broad bands, and contains vascular slits filled with extravasated erythrocytes. The diagnosis of Kaposi's sarcoma in very early skin lesions may be extremely difficult as little more may be seen than a few irregular dilated vascular channels in the mid dermis and a mild inflammatory cell infiltrate.

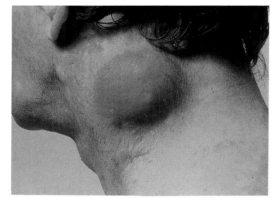

Extranodal lymphoma in the neck

Non-Hodgkins lymphoma

Extranodal disease is common and affects the central nervous system, bone marrow, and gastrointestinal tract. The diagnosis should also be considered in patients with weight loss, constitutional symptoms, and anaemia. The tumours originate from B cells, are of high or intermediate grade, and generally respond poorly to cytotoxic drugs. Squamous carcinomas of the mouth and anorectum have been described in homosexual men with antibodies to HIV. Human papillomavirus may play a part.

The opportunistic infections

The organisms responsible for the opportunistic infections occurring in patients with AIDS are unusual pathogens. Most of the infections are due to reactivation of latent organisms in the host or, in some cases, ubiquitous organisms to which we are continually exposed. The infections are often difficult to diagnose because conventional serological tests are unhelpful. Treatment often suppresses rather than eradicates the organisms. Relapses are therefore common, and continuous treatment with drugs, which may cause side effects, may be necessary.

Three main organ systems are affected—the respiratory system, the gastrointestinal tract, and the central nervous system. In addition, patients may present with a history of night sweats, chronic ill health, fevers, or weight loss.

Pulmonary complications

Pneumocystis carinii pneumonia is the commonest life threatening opportunistic infection in patients who progress from chronic HIV infection to AIDS. The presentation is subacute and malaise, fatigue, weight loss, and shortness of breath often develop during several weeks. Typical retrosternal or subcostal chest discomfort associated with increasing shortness of breath, a dry cough, and fever finally cause the patient to seek help. The chest x ray at presentation may be normal or show bilateral fine infiltrates, which are typically perihilar. The arterial oxygen tension is usually depressed, and the carbon monoxide transfer factor, when available, is low and may be the earliest detectable abnormality. The diagnosis is confirmed by cytological examination of induced sputum or by fibreoptic bronchoscopy and bronchial lavage. Transbronchial biopsy is now performed less often. Bronchoscopy can exclude other causes of

Chest radiograph of patient with typical appearances of *Pneumocystis carinii* pneumonia

Effect on respiratory system—typical results from bronchoscopy series

Condition	Percentage
Pneumocystis carinii pneumonia	70
Cytomegalovirus	15
Kaposi's sarcoma	5
Bacterial infection (pneumococcal, caused by *Haemophilus influenzae*, or mycobacterial (atypical or caused by *M tuberculosis*)	
Miscallaneous	5

Gastrointestinal complication of AIDS

Complications	Causes
Retrosternal discomfort and dysphagia	Candidiasis Cytomegalovirus (CMV) Herpes simplex virus (HSV)
Diarrhoea, weight loss, and malabsorption	Unknown—enteropathy Cryptosporidiosis, *Isospora belli*, and microsporidial infection CMV/HSV Mycobacteria Enteric bacteria—salmonella, campylobacter Neoplasia
Hepatitis and cholestasis	Mycobacteria CMV Drug induced Cryptosporidium
Perianal ulceration	HSV ?CMV
Neoplasia and miscellaneous	Kaposi's sarcoma Lymphoma Hairy leucoplakia Recalcitrant anorectal warts ? Squamous oral/anal carcinoma

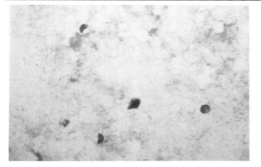

Cysts of cryptosporidium (modified Ziehl-Neelsen stain)

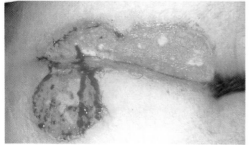

Severe mucocutaneous herpes simplex virus infection

pneumonia or coexistent infection such as cytomegalovirus, mycobacteria, and fungi.

Pyogenic bacterial causes of pneumonia should always be considered, particularly as its presentation may be atypical. The radiological appearances may include diffuse infiltrates as well as the more typical focal or lobar patterns. Another cause of diffuse abnormality is lymphocytic interstitial pneumonitis, first described in paediatric AIDS and now recognised in adults.

Infection with *Mycobacterium tuberculosis* may also occur. Pulmonary tuberculosis does not constitute a diagnosis of AIDS. The downward trend of reported cases of tuberculosis has slowed in the United States at the same rate as the HIV epidemic has grown. Pulmonary tuberculosis seems to appear in chronic HIV infection earlier than the atypical mycobacterial infections that complicate the severe immune depression of AIDS.

Gastrointestinal and hepatic complications

Retrosternal discomfort and dysphagia—oral and oesophageal candidiasis is the commonest cause of dysphagia or retrosternal discomfort. Oral candidiasis alone does not fulfil the criteria for AIDS. Oesophageal infection is best shown by culture or biopsy at endoscopy, although plaques of *Candida albicans* can often be seen during a barium swallow. Ulceration may be focal or diffuse. Cytomegalovirus and herpes simplex virus may both cause a similar pattern of ulceration in the oesophagus (and also may affect the stomach and duodenum). It may be difficult to differentiate between them by barium studies.

Diarrhoea, malabsorption, and weight loss—Diarrhoea is a common symptom of patients with chronic HIV infection, with or without other manifestations of AIDS. In many cases a cause is not found. Symptomatic treatment is all there is to offer. Enteropathy with villous atrophy and malabsorption has been described.

Cryptosporidium is a coccidian protozoal parasite and probably the commonest pathogen isolated from patients with AIDS who have diarrhoea. It is the commonest of the protozoal causes of diarrhoea, which also include *Isospora belli* and microsporidia. In immunocompetent human hosts cryptosporidium produces a transient diarrhoeal illness. In people infected with HIV it can cause transient, intermittent, or persistent diarrhoea, ranging from loose stools to watery diarrhoea, colic, and severe fluid and electrolyte loss. Oocysts (4–5 µm) can be found in stools. If direct smears of unconcentrated faecal samples stained with iodine or modified acid fast stains fail to show the oocysts the samples should be concentrated. The diagnosis should not be discounted without examining multiple specimens.

Cytomegalovirus and herpes simplex virus can cause focal or diffuse ulceration of the gut, from the mouth to the anus. Herpes simplex virus most commonly causes mucocutaneous lesions at the upper and the lower ends of the gastrointestinal tract, whereas cytomegalovirus may mimic inflammatory bowel disease.

Atypical mycobacteria of the avium intracellular complex are ubiquitous organisms that have little virulence for the immunocompetent host. Disseminated infection of several organs occurs in patients with AIDS. Gastrointestinal infection may be associated with fever, weight loss, diarrhoea, and malabsorption. Diagnosis can be made by acid fast staining of the stool or biopsy material, or both, or culture of blood or tissue. *Mycobacterium tuberculosis* infection of the bowel does occur, but is less common. *Campylobacter* and *Salmonella* species infections may cause diarrhoea, but the latter more commonly presents as a fever of unknown origin with bacteraemia.

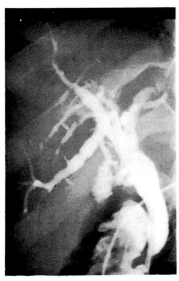

Dilated common bile duct with stricture at lower end and irregularities of extrahepatic and intrahepatic ducts

Hepatitis and cholestasis—Hepatitis in patients with AIDS may present as fever, abdominal pain, and hepatomegaly, and liver function test results, particularly raised alkaline phosphatase activity, may be abnormal. If ultrasound does not show dilated bile ducts, needle biopsy often shows granulomatous hepatitis, usually caused by atypical mycobacteria rather than *M tuberculosis*. The herpes viruses may also occasionally cause hepatitis as part of a disseminated infection. When multiple drugs are being taken, drug induced hepatitis must always be considered.

Acalculous cholecystis and cholangitis show an endoscopic retrograde cholangiographic picture similar to that of primary sclerosing cholangitis, with strictures and dilation of the biliary tree. Cryptosporidium and cytomegalovirus have been shown or isolated and are implicated as a cause of this syndrome.

Neurological complications

Chronic HIV infection is associated with several syndromes affecting the nervous system, in addition to the transient meningoencephalitis, myelopathy, and peripheral neuropathy of acute infection. These neurological diseases are believed to be due to the direct or indirect effects of HIV and not to opportunistic infection. AIDS related dementia (HIV encephalopathy) has been estimated to occur in 10–40% of patients with symptomatic disease. At necropsy up to 90% of patients dying of AIDS have chronic subcortical encephalitis characterised by infected macrophages and microglial cells that fuse to form multinucleate giant cells. There is also patchy demyelination and astrogliosis.

The clinical features are characterised by cognitive and behavioural changes that include memory loss, apathy, and impaired concentration and attention. Neurological examination may show hyperreflexia, hypertonia, and frontal release signs. Computed tomography or magnetic resonance imaging often show cerebral atrophy and non-specific changes in the white matter. The cerebrospinal fluid findings are non-specific. Opportunistic infections, intracranial mass lesions, metabolic encephalopathy, and neurosyphilis should be excluded.

HIV infection is also implicated in vacuolar myelopathy affecting primarily the posterior and lateral spinal cord, meningitis, and the following neuropathies: axonal sensory, chronic inflammatory demyelinating, and mononeuropathies. Cytomegalovirus infection may produce a polyradiculopathy.

The nervous system is also affected by opportunistic infection and tumour. Cerebral toxoplasmosis is the commonest cause of intracranial mass lesions and usually presents with focal symptoms and signs.

Rough incidence of conditions in patients with neurological complications	
Central nervous system (CNS)	Percentage
Viral infections	
AIDS related dementia	16
HIV related meningitis	13
CMV retinitis	5
CMV encephalitis	2
Progressive multifocal leucoencephalopathy	0·5
Vacuolar myelopathy	4*
Intracranial mass lesions	
Cerebral toxoplasmosis	14
Primary CNS lymphoma	4
Undefined mass lesions	3
Lymphoma	1
Peripheral nervous system	
Sensory neuropathy	16
Inflammatory demyelinating neuropathy	6
Cranial neuropathies	2
Multiple mononeuropathies	1
Polyradiculopathy	2
Miscellaneous	
Cryptococcal meningitis	6
Neurosyphilis	0·5
Metabolic encephalopathy	3
Cerebrovascular accident	0·5

* May be as high as 20% at necropsy.

Treatment

Zidovudine is a nucleoside analogue that has been shown to decrease mortality, the incidence of opportunistic infections, and constitutional symptoms in patients with symptomatic disease. It inhibits HIV replication by inhibiting the reverse transcriptase enzyme. It suppresses P24 antigenaemia and produces a modest, usually transient, increase in CD4 cell count. However, it causes

Protozoal opportunistic infections

Infection	Drug	Duration	Side effects	Comments
Pneumocystic carinii pneumonia				
Treatment	Co-trimoxazole (trimethoprim component 20 mg/kg/day) intravenusly for 14 days then orally	14–21 days	Nausea, fever, rash, bone marrow suspension	80% of patients will respond to treatment
	or pentamidine isethionate 4 mg/kg/day or pentamidine mesylate 2·5 mg/kg/day, both as a slow intravenous infusion	14–21 days	Hypotension, hypoglycaemia, renal failure, hepatitis, bone marrow suppression	
	or nebulised pentamidine isethionate (8 mg/kg/day)	14–21 days	Bronchospasm, metallic taste	Patients may prefer as no injection and fewer side effects
Maintenance	Co-trimoxazole 960 mg a day or on alternate days or pyrimethamine 25 mg and sulfadoxine 500 mg a week or dapsone 100 mg a week or nebulised pentamidine isethionate 8 mg/kg every 2–4 weeks	Indefinite	Usually minimal	Exact dose or frequency not yet established
Toxoplasmosis	Pyrimethamine 50 mg/day orally and either sulphadiazine 4–6 mg/day orally or clindamycin 600 mg four times/day	Indefinite	Rash, nausea, bone marrow suppression	Doses usually halved during maintenance
		Indefinite		
Cryptosporidiosis	Spiramycin 1 g four times/day	14 days		
	or erythromycin 500 mg four times a day	14 days	Nausea, rash	No treatment is of proved value
	or clindamycin 300 mg four times a day and quinine 250 mg four times a day	14 days		
Isosporiasis	Co-trimoxazole 960 mg four times a day orally	Indefinite	See above	

Viral opportunistic infections

Infection	Drug	Duration	Side effects	Comments
Herpes simplex				
Treatment	Acyclovir 200 mg 5 times a day orally or 5–10 mg/kg 8 hourly intravenously	10–14 days		
Prophylaxis	Acyclovir 200 mg four times a day	Indefinite		May be possible to reduce frequency
Cytomegalovirus				
Treatment	Ganciclovir 5 mg/kg twice a day	14–21 days	Anaemia, neutropenia	Marrow suppression potentiated with zidovudine
Prophylaxis	Ganciclovir 2·5–5 mg/kg/day	Indefinite	Anaemia, neutropenia	

Fungal opportunistic infections

Infection	Drug	Duration	Side effects	Comments
Candidiasis				
Local treatment	Nystatin oral suspension or pastilles, miconazole oral gel, or amphotericin lozenges all 4–6 times a day	As required		Relapse common, many patients require systemic treatment
Systemic treatment	Ketoconazole 200–400 mg a day orally or fluconazole 50–200 mg/day	Indefinite	Nausea, hepatitis, thrombocytopenia	Relapse common on cessation of treatment
Maintenance	Fluconazole 50–100 mg/day or alternate days	6 weeks Indefinite	Nausea	
Cryptococcosis	Amphotericin B 0·3 mg/kg/day and flucytosine 150 mg/kg/day in 4 doses	6 weeks	Nausea, vomiting, rash, bone marrow suppression, renal damage, hypocalcaemia	Relapse may occur, maintenance needed
	or fluconazole 200–400 mg/day	6 weeks	Nausea	

Dideoxynucleosides

T

5'
HOCH2 O
4   1   Thymidine
  3' 2
OH

T

5'
HOCH2 O
4   1   3'–Azido–3'–deoxythmidin
   3' 2
N3

C

5'
HOCH2 O
4   1   2'–deoxycytidine
  3' 2
OH

C

5'
HOCH2 O
4   1   2'–3' dideoxycytidine
  3' 2
H

gastrointestinal side effects and, more important, its use is associated with anaemia and neutropenia that often necessitate dose reduction or interruption of treatment. Long term complications include myopathy and the emergence of viral strains with reduced sensitivity.

Other 2'3' dideoxynucleoside analogues such as 2'3' dideoxycytidine (ddC) and 2'3' dideoxyinosine (ddI) are being evaluated in comparative studies, either alone or in combination with zidovudine, in patients with symptomatic disease. Both cause peripheral neuropathy at high doses.

Basic research is delivering more specific and less empirical antiviral drugs that are being evaluated in early trials. Recombinant CD4 and CD4 linked to an immunoglobulin (immunoadhesin, which prolongs the half life) block infection of cells, cell fusion, and other mechanisms by which cells are killed in HIV infection. Characterisation of viral enzymes that process viral proteins, such as HIV protease, has facilitated the design of specific inhibitors soon to be assessed in people.

Despite the advances in producing antiviral drugs, treatment is still directed largely at the main complications of the disease. Conventional cytotoxic drugs and radiotherapy are used for Kaposi's sarcoma. Alfa interferon has also been used. All induce remission in some cases, but none alter median survival. Some regimens carry increased risks of opportunistic infection and side effects that affect the quality of life considerably.

There have been important advances in managing opportunistic infections with alternative treatments, such as nebulised pentamidine for *P carinii* pneumonia, the now widespread use of ganciclovir and phosphonoformate for cytomegalovirus infections, and new systemic antifungal agents such as fluconazole.

The improvement in survival of patients with symptomatic disease that has been seen in the past two years has been due to the introduction of zidovudine, earlier diagnosis and treatment of complications, and the extended use of antimicrobial prophylaxis, particularly for *P carinii* pneumonia.

Prevention and control

Prevention and control
- Surveillance
- Counselling and health education
- (a) Screening of people and
       donated blood
  (b) Heat treatment of
       blood products
- Protection of health care staff

As no cure or vaccine is currently available, our main weapon is prevention and control. An "information vaccine" is required. In any epidemic an accurate appreciation of the size of the problem and how it is changing is essential. With HIV infection this can be achieved by counting the number of patients with AIDS and monitoring the prevalence of antibody to HIV in low and high risk populations.

Of fundamental importance is good and accurate health education for those at low risk and those at high risk. People who may have been exposed are advised not to donate blood, organs, or semen, and to modify their sexual behaviour to avoid practices that are particularly likely to transmit the virus. The screening of blood donors for antibody to HIV and the heat treatment of blood products have virtually eliminated the risk to recipients.

GENITAL WARTS AND MOLLUSCUM CONTAGIOSUM

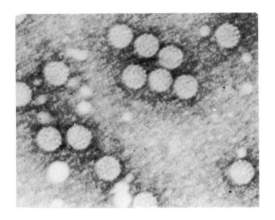

Even though genital warts (condyloma acuminatum) are commonly seen in departments of genitourinary medicine (about 84 000 cases a year, 12% of all cases seen) many more cases are diagnosed and treated by general practitioners, surgeons, gynaecologists, and dermatologists. Not only are warts common but they are difficult and time consuming to treat.

They are caused by a small DNA virus, a papillomavirus belonging to the papovavirus group, which cannot be cultured. Genital warts differ from skin warts histologically and antigenically. Genital warts are nearly always transmitted by sexual contact; autoinoculation from hand to genitals is unusual. Infants and young children may develop laryngeal papillomas due to infection from maternal genital warts at delivery. The infectivity of sexually acquired warts is about 60%; the incubation period is long, varying from two weeks to eight months (mean three months).

Clinical features

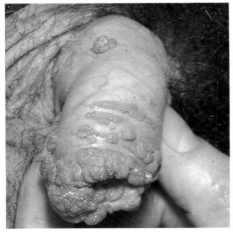

Genital warts are often asymptomatic and painless. Patients may give a history of suddenly noticing them or noticing them only once their sexual contact has acquired them. Women are more likely to be unaware of warts because it is harder for them to examine their genitalia. Warts flourish in warm, moist conditions, particularly if a discharge or other infections are present.

Warts may be solitary but are usually multiple by the time the patient attends for consultation. In men they may be found on the glans and shaft of the penis, prepuce, fraenum and coronal sulcus, urethral meatus, scrotum, anus, and rectum. Even though anal warts usually occur after anal intercourse they may occur without this. In women the commonest site of infection is the introitus and vulva, but warts may also affect the vagina and (as flat warts) the cervix. Other infected sites may be the perineum, anus, and rectum.

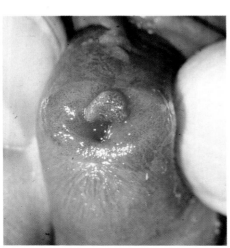
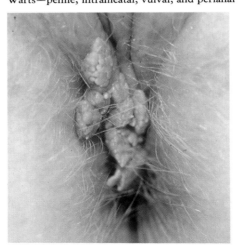
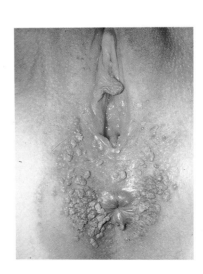

Warts—penile, intrameatal, vulval, and perianal

Diagnosis

Complications

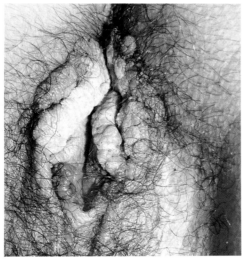

Massive warts in pregnancy

Treatment

Genital warts and molluscum contagiosum

Genital warts are one of the few sexually transmitted conditions that are diagnosed solely from their clinical features. Diagnosis is not usually difficult but the differential diagnosis of condylomata lata of secondary syphilis, molluscum contagiosum, sebaceous cysts, and benign and malignant tumours should be remembered. Warts may often herald other sexually transmitted diseases or infections. For example, one third of women attending departments of genitourinary medicine with genital warts have one or more additional diseases diagnosed concurrently. All women with genital warts, even in the absence of any other symptoms, must have a full set of microbiological tests performed to exclude, at least, infection with *Candida albicans, Trichomonas vaginalis, Neisseria gonorrhoea,* and also, if possible, *Gardnerella vaginalis* and *Chlamydia trachomatis.* Heterosexual and homosexual men with penile warts should have urethral tests for gonorrhoea and non-gonococcal urethritis, even if they are asymptomatic. Likewise, homosexuals with anal warts should have proctoscopy performed to exclude the presence of additional warts within the rectum as well as other rectal diseases such as gonorrhoea. Finally, serological tests for syphilis should be carried out in both men and women. Contact tracing of regular sexual partners must be undertaken as well as full microbiological investigations.

Complications of genital warts are rare. Occasionally they may increase alarmingly in size during pregnancy and appear as large cauliflower like masses. In men similar giant benign but destructive warts (Buschke–Lowenstein tumour) may occur on the penis or existing small ones may rapidly become enlarged. Malignant transformation of vulval, cervical, penile, and anal warts has been reported. As yet no case-control studies confirming the association between human papillomavirus infection and carcinoma of the cervix have been undertaken.

Flat warts on the cervix are not usually apparent to the naked eye. Their possible association with cervical intraepithelial neoplasia means that in ideal circumstances all regular female consorts of men with warts, and all women with vulval warts, should undergo colposcopy to exclude cervical warts. The present lack of proof that malignant change does occur means that a more pragmatic approach is to encourage all women attending clinics to have cytology performed every year.

Initial treatment is usually with locally applied caustic agents. It is usual to start with podophyllin—a cytotoxic agent—which should be applied to the lesions in strengths of 10% or 25% in industrial spirit and repeated at least twice or even three times a week. Being an irritating substance it can cause bad burns. Patients must therefore be told to wash it off three to four hours after application. Patients may often want to apply podophyllin themselves but this is undesirable, since they may be overzealous in their justifiable desire to get rid of their warts and apply the substance too often, without washing it off, on the basis that "if it hurts it must be doing me good." Severe systemic effects of peripheral neuropathy, coma, and hypokalaemia can follow application of large quantities. Podophyllotoxin 0·5% has less severe side effects and could be used by the patient to apply at home. If podophyllin applied regularly is ineffective after two to three weeks the more caustic agent glacial trichloroacetic acid 50–100% may be used, again with great caution. This agent is more often used for hyperkeratotic warts but even so these warts are often resistant and electrocautery or cryotherapy will be needed. Cautery or surgical excision should be considered at an earlier stage if the warts are particularly large or numerous. The clinical course of warts, particularly their ability to regress spontaneously and reappear, has made other treatment regimens—such as vaccines, fluorouracil, and interferon—difficult to assess.

Genital warts and molluscum contagiosum

Approaches to the treatment of genital warts

Site or type of warts	Start	1 week	2 weeks	3 weeks	4 weeks
Few, small, and soft	10–25% Podophyllin	→————→	————→	Trichloroethanoic acid	Cryotherapy electrocautery
Extensive, multiple, vegetations	10–25% Podophyllin or Trichloroethanoic acid	————→	Surgical excision		
Hyperkeratotic	Trichloroethanoic acid	————→	Electrocautery diathermy		
Intrameatal	10% Podophyllin	————→	Electrocautery cryotherapy		
Solitary, large, discrete	Electrocautery diathermy, excision				
Cervical	Colposcopy, cryotherapy, laser				
Pregnancy	None—unless discrete small vaginal or vulval, then use trichloroethanoic acid/cryotherapy-? electrocautery				

Treatment of warts outside departments of genitourinary medicine

- Sexual and genitourinary history

- Exclude a concurrent sexually transmitted disease

- Trace regular sexual contacts

Molluscum contagiosum

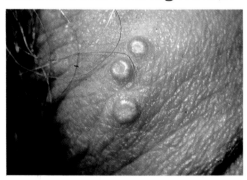

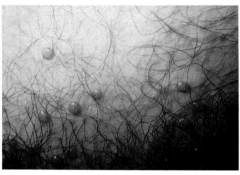

During pregnancy it is best to offer no treatment. Podophyllin is contraindicated in view of its toxicity and possible mutagenic action, and the warts usually diminish in size once pregnancy has ended. Withholding treatment in this way has to be weighed against the possible development of laryngeal papilloma in the neonate. This is rare and does not justify the use of a cytotoxic drug during pregnancy. Trichloracetic acid may be used if the lesions are discrete and small and occur on the vaginal wall or vulva. Alternatively, cryotherapy or electrocautery may be offered. Occasionally caesarean section is necessary if the warts are likely to obstruct labour.

Doctors treating genital warts outside sexually transmitted disease clinics should remember, firstly, that an accurate and detailed sexual and genitourinary history is needed; secondly, that concurrent sexually acquired conditions should be excluded; and, thirdly, that contact tracing must be carried out.

Molluscum contagiosum may be transmitted sexually but this is not the only route. It is a contagious viral condition which may be spread by close bodily contact, clothing, or towels. Transmission (outbreaks) is possible in swimming pools, sauna baths, schools, after massage, and between siblings. The agent causing molluscum contagiosum is one of the pox viruses and has a variable incubation period of two to twelve weeks. Only 3400 cases a year are diagnosed in clinics; far more cases are probably seen by general practitioners and dermatologists.

Clinical features—The lesions of molluscum contagiosum are characteristic. The pearly white umbilicated papules appear in the genital area (penis, scrotum, vulva, perineum, abdomen, and thighs), but if transmission is non-sexual they may also be found in any part of the body but particularly on the arms, face, eyelids, and scalp. The lesions are usually small (2–5 mm in diameter).

Diagnosis is usually based on the clinical appearance since the virus cannot be grown successfully. Material expressed from the centre of lesions shows viral inclusions on Giemsa stain or on electron microscopy. Since the condition may be sexually transmitted other infections similarly spread should be excluded if the patient's history or the site of the lesions (proximity to genital area) suggests that this could be the route of infection.

Treatment is by applying phenol on the end of a sharpened stick to the central umbilicated core of the lesions. This may need to be repeated several times. Alternatively electrocautery or cryotherapy may be used.

GENITAL INFESTATIONS

Pediculosis pubis

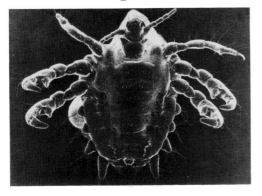

Pediculosis pubis is caused by the pubic louse, *Phthirus pubis*, which is a different species from that causing head and body louse infestation (pediculosis capitis and corporis). The insect is small and round (1–2 mm long) and has three sets of legs. The adult adheres not only to pubic hair but also to other hairy areas (perenium, thighs, abdomen, axillas, eyebrows, and eyelashes) and is a blood sucker. The female lays eggs (nits) at the base of the hairs and these usually hatch within seven days. The adult louse is transferred from person to person during close bodily contact. Since lice do not leave the host the condition is not spread by wearing or sleeping in infested clothing or sheets. The patient may complain of irritation. Sometimes the condition is asymptomatic and the patient may be horrified to find the adult louse or nits on the body.

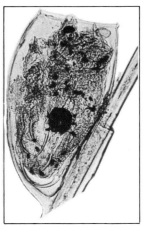

Diagnosis is usually based on clinical appearances alone. A hand lens is useful during the examination and a suspected louse on a hair may be removed and viewed under the low power microscope. Bluish grey macules occasionally occur on the abdomen, buttocks, or thighs at the site of the bites. As the condition is usually sexually acquired a full genitourinary and sexual history must be taken and the patient examined for other sexually transmitted diseases. Blood must also be taken for syphilis serology.

Treatment—1% gamma benzene hexachloride powder (Gammexane) or 0·5% Malathion should be applied to all the hairy areas apart from the scalp. The patient should not wash this off for 24 hours, after which a bath should be taken. Usually one application is enough, but a heavy infestation will necessitate further treatment within 7–10 days. Alternatively 1% gamma benzene hexachloride can be used as a cream or lotion (Lorexane, Quellada) or Carbaryl as 0·5% lotion (Carylderm, Clinicide, Suleo-c, Derbac Shampoo). There is no need to wash the patient's clothes and bed linen. Sexual partners should also be seen and treated, as well as family contacts who could be infected. Shaving of body hair is not necessary.

Gamma benzene hexachloride should not be used in pregnant women since it is lipid soluble and can be stored in body fat and appear in breast milk.

Management of pediculosis pubis

0 hours	Gamma benzene hexachloride 1% – powder (Gammexane) – cream (Lorexane) – lotion (Quellada) or 0·5% Malathion or 0·5% Carbaryl
24 hours	Bath Sexual and family contacts seen and treated
7 days	Repeat treatment if necessary

Sexually transmitted disease

Genital infestations

Scabies

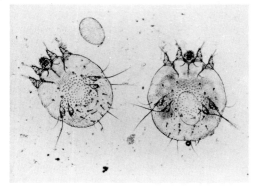

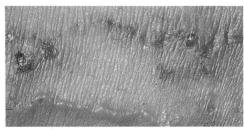

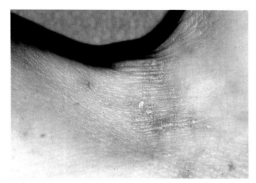

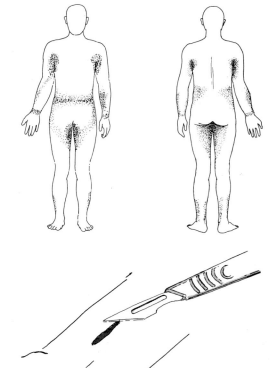

Infestation is caused by the mite *Sarcoptes scabiei*. The clinical features of scabies are caused by the female burrowing into the uppermost layer of the skin (stratum corneum) and laying eggs and defecating. The female is about twice the size (0·3 mm long) of the male and can just be seen by the naked eye as a black dot (mouth parts) at the distal part of the burrow. Infestation usually occurs as a result of close physical, but not necessarily sexual, contact. This needs to be reasonably prolonged since the insect moves slowly, at 25 mm a minute. Outbreaks of non-sexually acquired scabies may occur among schoolchildren and within whole households or long stay hospitals.

Symptoms are first noticed two to six weeks after infestation. Reinfection may give rise to symptoms within a few hours. The patient complains of itching, which is often unbearable, intractable, and worse at night when the body is warm. The sites of itching and burrows bear no relation to the mode of transmission. Thus lesions may often be found in the clefts of fingers and on the wrists and elbows as well as on the genitals. On examination the burrows may be the typical sinuous scaling reddish grey lesions (5–15 mm long), sometimes with small vesicles at their end. Scratching may, however, alter their appearance, with excoriation, ulceration, crusting, and bleeding; on the penis and scrotum they may appear as red papules. Associated rashes may also be found in sites distant from the actual burrows—in particular erythematous urticarial papules in the armpits, abdominal wall, and the anterior and posterior aspects of the upper thighs. In some cases indurated nodules, eczematous changes, and secondary infection with pustule formation may occur.

Diagnosis is based on the clinical history and examination and may be confirmed by finding the mite. This is achieved by scraping the top off the whole length of a burrow (from distal to proximal end) with a scalpel, putting the material on a slide with 10% potassium hydroxide solution, and looking for the mite under the microscope. As with pediculosis pubis, if the history suggests sexual transmission other sexually transmitted diseases must be excluded.

Treatment—Scabies is treated by the application of 25% benzyl benzoate solution to the whole body from the neck downwards, not forgetting the soles of the feet. This is best applied using a broad paintbrush. Unless this is carried out in a clinic the patient will need help from a relative or friend to achieve total coverage. Treatment should be repeated 24 hours later. On the third day (after 48 hours) the patient should take a bath. Alternatively 1% gamma benzene hexachloride cream or lotion or 0·5% malathion can be applied to the whole body. Patients should be told that the initial itching may persist for several weeks despite successful treatment with either preparation. Unless this explanation is given patients may equate the symptoms with continuing infection, retreat themselves, and run the risk of a chemical dermatitis. Sexual contacts should be seen if sexual transmission is suspected; if the condition was not acquired by this route other members of the family or school friends will need to be treated. When contacts are seen they may be asymptomatic but should be treated since they may be incubating the disease.

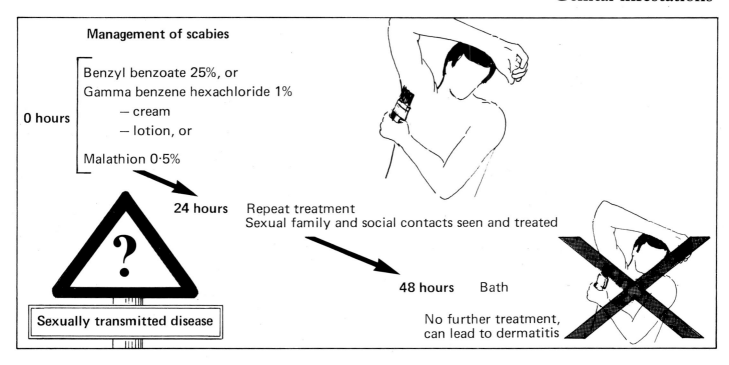

Management of scabies

0 hours — Benzyl benzoate 25%, or
Gamma benzene hexachloride 1%
— cream
— lotion, or
Malathion 0·5%

24 hours — Repeat treatment
Sexual family and social contacts seen and treated

48 hours — Bath

Sexually transmitted disease

No further treatment, can lead to dermatitis

Tinea cruris

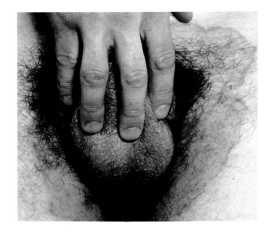

Tinea cruris is a common skin condition, particularly in men. If limited to the groin area it is caused by one of two fungi—*Trichophyton rubrum* or *Epidermophyton floccosum*. The patient may complain of an irritating rash, particularly in the groin. When patients attend a department of genitourinary medicine with this condition they may be extremely distraught because they fear that the condition is sexually acquired or even, having read about rashes, fear that it could be due to syphilis. The same type of patient consulting doctors outside the clinics may regard the condition as no more than a "sweat rash."

The rash has a scaly, marginated, erythematous appearance, the edges of which are occasionally vesicular or pustular. It needs to be differentiated from a seborrhoeic or contact dermatitis, psoriasis, and candidiasis. The diagnosis is based on the clinical history and appearance and may be confirmed by mixing scrapings of the lesions with 10% potassium hydroxide solution and viewing them under a normal microscope, when mycelium can be seen. The fungi may be cultured on Sabouraud's medium. Treatment with benzoic acid compound ointment *BPC* (Whitfield's ointment half strength) is cheap and highly effective. Alternatively imidazole derivatives can be applied as a cream (clotrimazole, miconazole, econazole). This is applied once or twice daily until the lesions disappear and should be continued for a further one to two weeks to avoid reappearance. Newer imidazole derivatives may be given, and in severe resistant or relapsing cases griseofulvin may have to be used, at a dosage of 500 mg once or twice daily for six weeks.

Management

Normally: Benzoic acid compound ointment BPC (Whitfield's ointment ½ strength) twice daily, continue for 1–2 weeks after resolution
Clotrimazole, miconazole, or econazole

Resistant/relapsing: Griseofulvin, 500 mg once-twice a day for six weeks

GENITAL SKIN AND OTHER CONDITIONS

Lichen sclerosus et atrophicus
Lichen planus
Psoriasis and dermatitis
Dermatitis
Trauma
Lymphocele
Peyronie's disease

Several skin and other conditions may affect the genital area but are not sexually transmitted. Because of their anatomical site patients with these conditions seek medical advice in the fear that they have acquired a sexually transmitted disease.

Lichen sclerosus et atrophicus

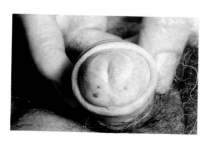

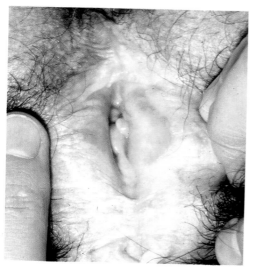

Lichen sclerosus et atrophicus is a rare disease that may occur in any age group but usually in those aged 30–60 years. The aetiology is unknown. The skin in the affected areas is atrophic, with white plaques and eventual contraction of tissues. When localised to the male genitals the condition is called balanitis xerotica obliterans. In men the major sites affected are the glans penis, urethral meatus with extension into the terminal urethra, and the prepuce. In women the changes are found on the vulva, vaginal introitus, clitoris, perineum, and anus.

Clinical features—Men with this condition may present with penile pain and irritation, urethral discharge, and in the later stages of the disease phimosis and urinary obstruction. Women may notice itching of the vulva, sometimes associated with superficial dyspareunia. The dyspareunia may also be due to lesions on the vaginal introitus. The condition should not be forgotten as one of the causes of persistent pruritus vulvae.

On examination white plaques may be seen on the glans and prepuce, often encircling the end of the foreskin, which may be difficult to retract. The urethral meatus may also be surrounded with a small collar of white tissue extending a small distance up the urethra so that the first centimetre is pipe stem hard and the meatus very small in size. In women the same type of plaques may be found on the vulva, and the skin may often appear thin, with a parchment quality, and shiny. These skin changes may affect other areas of the body. In some cases erythema, purpura, excoriations, blister formation, and pigmentary changes may also be seen.

Diagnosis and treatment—The diagnosis should be confirmed by biopsy and histology. The aim of treatment is both to relieve the symptoms and to slow down the disease process. This may often be achieved by the application of a potent topical corticosteroid cream twice a day. In addition the skin may be moisturised and softened by the use of aqueous cream *BP* as a soap substitute and moisturising cream. Long term follow up is recommended since the lesions, particularly the phimosis and meatal narrowing, may progress and require dilatation, meatotomy, or circumcision. Neoplastic changes (squamous cell carcinoma) of the lesions may occur later.

Lichen planus

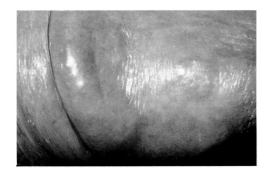

Lichen planus affects the genital area and other parts of the body and may present with mauvish papules or plaques. Usually the patient complains of itching at the site of the lesions, which occur on the glans penis, shaft, foreskin, scrotum, vulva, and perianal areas. The lesions may be papular or annular and are often white, particularly if situated in moist parts of the body. They may also be found in extragenital areas such as the arms, flexor aspects of the wrists, legs, and buccal epithelium. The disease is eventually self limiting but some relief can be obtained with a topical corticosteroid cream or ointment.

Psoriasis and dermatitis

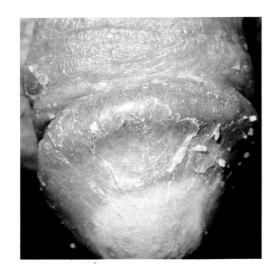

Both psoriasis and dermatitis may affect the genital area either alone or in conjunction with widespread disease elsewhere. The lesions of psoriasis may be found on the penis, scrotum, vulva, groins, perineum, and perianal areas. These are often similar to the scaly red psoriasiform lesions found in other parts of the body. They may, however, lose their scales if present in moist parts of the genitalia and appear red and shiny. The condition has to be differentiated from tinea cruris, candidiasis, lichen planus, keratodermia blennorrhagia, erythroplasia, and seborrhoeic or contact dermatitis. In relation to the sexually transmitted diseases the most important condition that may look the same is the scaly papular rash of secondary syphilis. The presence of psoriasis in non-genital areas and the nails will help to exclude syphilis, however, though patients with psoriasis may also have syphilis. Psoriasis and dermatitis are not contagious but in patients presenting with skin conditions affecting the genital area it is essential to bear in mind that such conditions could be sexually acquired and to examine the entire surface of the skin.

The treatment of psoriasis affecting the genital region is the same as that for the condition in general—with coal tar preparations and corticosteroid ointments.

Dermatitis

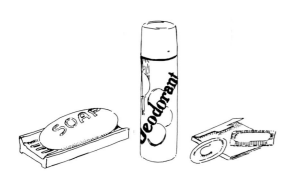

There are two common types of dermatitis of the genitalia—seborrhoeic or contact. Seborrhoeic dermatitis is only rarely localised to the genital area, and other areas such as the scalp, ears, chest, axillas, and back may be affected. The lesions are red and scaly and not well circumscribed. Again all skin areas must be examined. The condition is not related to any known precipitating factors and in this way differs from contact dermatitis. On careful questioning patients with contact dermatitis may relate their symptoms to the use of particular soaps, deodorants, forms of clothing, medicaments, and occasionally the sheath or to friction and trauma. They may complain of irritation possibly associated with swelling. Unless the patient is examined during the acute phase there will be little to see apart from mild erythema. Should the contact dermatitis continue, however, thickening and scaling of the skin may occur. Patch testing is likely to be needed to confirm the diagnosis if there is a possibility of an allergic contact dermatitis.

The symptomatic treatment of dermatitis is usually with topical corticosteroid preparations. In contact dermatitis the causative agent should be removed.

Genital skin and other conditions

Trauma

- **Deliberate** Atypical lesions

  Bizarre appearance

  Accessible to patient's hand

  Psychiatric assessment

- **Accidental** Atypical lesions

  Mechanical instruments

  Surgical repair
  (occasionally)

Several genital conditions, such as trauma, lymphocele, and Peyronie's disease, may be alarming both to the doctor and the patient. Trauma to the genitalia may be purposely or accidentally inflicted. Purposely self inflicted trauma (dermatitis artefacta) should be suspected when atypical lesions are present. They look bizarre, do not resemble any known condition, and are found in areas accessible to the patient's hand. The patient, who usually denies the aetiology, is often mentally unstable, and psychiatric assessment and help are needed.

The number of cases of accidental self inflicted genital trauma has risen in the last few years, because of the increased use of sexual aids and the more overt expression and possibilities for sadomasochistic sexual practices. These patients are not unstable. Trauma can follow anal intercourse using mechanical instruments, penile rings, or insertion of the whole forearm into the rectum. The reason for suspecting trauma is that the anal, rectal, and penile lesions tend to be atypical and unlike infective causes of ulceration, balanitis, etc. The lesions usually heal spontaneously but occasionally surgical repair is required.

Lymphocele

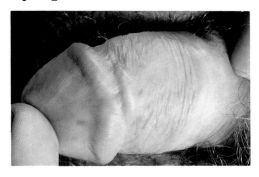

Lymphocele is a totally benign condition but very alarming to patients. The patient notices a cord-like swelling around the coroneal sulcus. It is sometimes accompanied by lymphangitis of the dorsum of the shaft. This may follow prolonged or particularly energetic sexual intercourse or masturbation, but this is by no means an essential prerequisite. The condition arises as a result of temporary obstruction of the lymphatics. No treatment is required, apart from reassurance and the explanation that it will resolve itself, which it does within a few days.

Peyronie's disease

Aetiology unknown

Pain and bending of penis

Spontaneous resolution

Surgery /steroids

Peyronie's disease is an alarming and distressing condition in which the patient first notices pain and permanent bending of the penis, particularly when erect. This is due to chronic fibrosis of the intercavernous septums of the penis. The condition may occur in association with Dupuytren's contracture. The aetiology is unknown. It usually occurs in middle aged men. On examination a hard ridge or lump of fibrous tissue may be felt on the dorsal aspect of the shaft of the penis and occasionally on the ventral and lateral aspect.

A few cases resolve spontaneously, which makes treatment claims difficult to assess. Surgical excision of the plaques is sometimes recommended, as are injections of the tissue with hydrocortisone.

Psychological effects

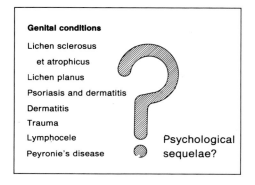

Genital conditions

Lichen sclerosus
   et atrophicus
Lichen planus
Psoriasis and dermatitis
Dermatitis
Trauma
Lymphocele
Peyronie's disease

Psychological sequelae?

Doctors treating patients with disfiguring lesions of the genitals should not forget the profound psychological sequelae that may be associated with them. Patients often do not show their concern and practitioners may need to take the initiative in discussing these aspects and giving reassurance. If this is not possible or the condition is permanent psychiatric support may be needed.

SYPHILIS: CLINICAL FEATURES

Extent of the problem

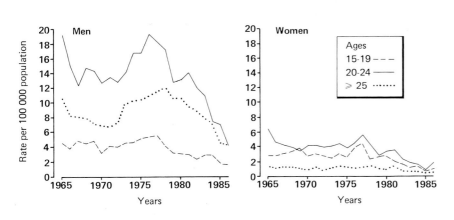

The advent of penicillin made a dramatic and rapid impact on the incidence of early infectious syphilis throughout the world in the late 1940s. The number of cases of syphilis seen in clinics is now less than a fifth of that seen during the peak just after the second world war (27 761). Rates for syphilis are higher in men than in women. This disparity is explained by the fact that in the past more than half of the male cases were acquired homosexually. The recent substantial decline could therefore indicate a change in behaviour among this group of men.

Classification

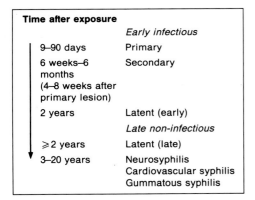

Time after exposure	
	Early infectious
9–90 days	Primary
6 weeks–6 months (4–8 weeks after primary lesion)	Secondary
2 years	Latent (early)
	Late non-infectious
≥2 years	Latent (late)
3–20 years	Neurosyphilis Cardiovascular syphilis Gummatous syphilis

Sites of primary syphilis

Genital	*Extragenital*
Shaft of penis	Lip
Coronal sulcus	Tongue
Glans penis	Mouth, tonsil, pharynx
Prepuce	Fingers
Fraenum	Eyelid
Urethral meatus	Nipple
Anal margin/canal	Any part of skin or
Rectum	mucous membranes
Labia minora/majora	
Fourchette	
Clitoris	
Vaginal wall	
Cervix	

Acquired syphilis has been classified traditionally into early infectious and late non-infectious stages. The arbitrary cut off point between these is usually two years.

Primary syphilis—The incubation period for primary syphilis is 9 to 90 days (mean 21 days). Lesions appear at the site of inoculation; these sites may sometimes be extragenital. The lesion is normally solitary and painless. It first appears as a red macule which progresses into a papule and finally ulcerates. This ulcer is usually round and clean with an indurated base and edges. Inguinal lymph nodes are moderately enlarged, rubbery, painless, and discrete. The primary lesions will heal within three to 10 weeks and may go unnoticed by the patient. Lesions on the cervix, rectum, anal canal, and margin may in particular be asymptomatic.

Secondary syphilis—The lesions of secondary syphilis usually occur four to eight weeks after the appearance of the primary lesion. In about one third of cases the primary lesion is still present. The lesions are generalised, affecting skin and mucous membranes.

The skin lesions are usually symmetrical and non-itchy. They can be macular, papular, papulosquamous, and very rarely pustular. The *macular* lesions are usually the first to appear as rose pink, rounded, discrete lesions (0·5–1 cm in diameter) on the shoulders, chest, back, abdomen, and arms. The *papular* lesions are coppery red and the same size as the macules. They may occur on the trunk, palms, arms, legs, soles, face, and genitalia. (Skin lesions are commonly a mixture of macular and papular (maculopapular).)

Syphilis: clinical features

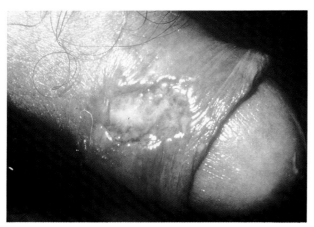
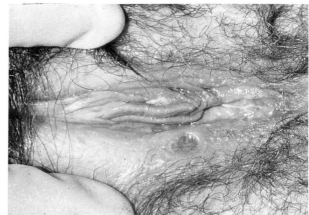

Primary chancre of penis and vulva

Lesions of secondary syphilis		
Skin:	Macular ⎫ maculopapular	
	Papular ⎭	
	Condylomata lata	
	Papulosquamous	
	Pustular	
Mucous membranes:	Erosions	

Clinical features of secondary syphilis	
Skin lesions	75–80%
Mucous membrane lesions	30%
Generalised lymphadenopathy	50–60%
Arthritis, arthralgia, periostitis	
Hepatitis	
Glomerulonephritis and nephrotic syndrome	Rare (<10%)
Iridocyclitis and choroidoretinitis	
Neurological disease (meningitis, cranial nerve palsies)	
Alopecia	

In warm opposed areas of the body (anus, labia) papular lesions can become large and coalesce to appear as large fleshy masses (condylomata lata). The *papulosquamous* lesions are found when scaling of the papules occurs and can be seen in association with straightforward papular lesions. If papulosquamous lesions occur on the palms or soles they are sometimes described as psoriasiform. *Pustular* lesions are rare and occur when the papular lesions undergo central necrosis. *Mucous membrane* lesions are shallow, painless erosions which usually appear in association with papular skin lesions and affect the mucous surface of lips, cheeks, tongue, fauces, pharynx and larynx, nose, vulva, vagina, glans penis, prepuce, and cervix. They have a greyish apperance and are sometimes described as "snail track" ulcers.

The lesions of skin and mucous membrane may be associated with non-specific constitutional symptoms of malaise, fever, anorexia, and generalised lymphadenopathy. The secondary stage is one of bacteriaemia, and any organ may show evidence of this—for example, hepatitis, iritis, meningitis, and optic neuritis with papilloedema.

Features of secondary syphilis: maculopapular rash on hands and chest and condylomata data

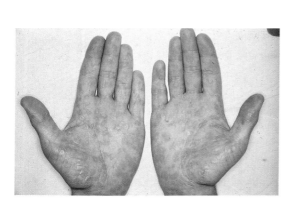

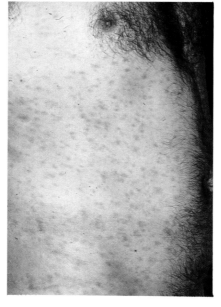
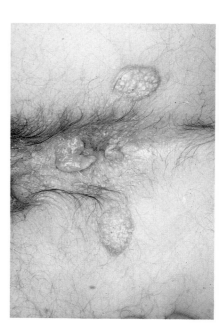

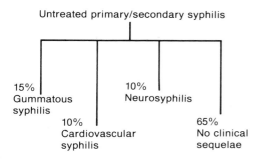

Untreated primary/secondary syphilis

15% Gummatous syphilis

10% Cardiovascular syphilis

10% Neurosyphilis

65% No clinical sequelae

Neurosyphilis

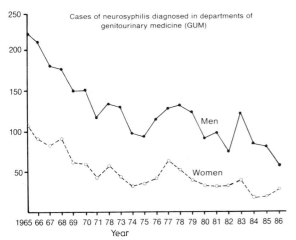

Cases of neurosyphilis diagnosed in departments of genitourinary medicine (GUM)

Latent syphilis—The latent period of syphilis follows the secondary stage. This latent period is divided into early and late. Early means that the disease has been present for less than two years and late for more than this time. The term latent means that there are no overt symptoms or signs of the disease and that the patient has never been treated. The condition is diagnosed from positive results to serological tests; no clinical evidence of early or late syphilis in any system; normal results on chest radiography and screening; and examination of cerebrospinal fluid to exclude cardiovascular syphilis or neurosyphilis. (Diagnosing syphilis is discussed in the next chapter.)

About 65% of patients with untreated syphilis will not develop late clinical sequelae of the disease. About 10% will develop neurological, 10% cardiovascular, and 15% gummatous lesions. Late syphilis is now rare.

Neurosyphilis is classified into asymptomatic, meningovascular, and parenchymatous (general paralysis of the insane and tabes dorsalis). The widespread use of antibiotics for other unrelated conditions has probably resulted in neurosyphilis which does not always fit the older classical clinical forms and descriptions.

Asymptomatic—As the name suggests, there are no neurological symptoms or signs and the diagnosis is based entirely on changes in the cerebrospinal fluid and serum.

Meningovascular disease can present at both early and late stages of syphilis. Patients can present with acute meningeal involvement during the secondary stages of the disease, often coinciding with the development of skin lesions. Headache is the main symptom. Signs of meningitis are found with third, sixth, and eighth cranial nerve involvement, papilloedema, and, rarely, homonymous hemianopia or hemiplegia. Late meningovascular syphilis presents less acutely but headaches may still be a presenting symptom. Cranial nerve palsies (third, sixth, seventh, and eighth) and pupillary abnormalities are seen. The pupils are small and unequal in size and react to accommodation but not light (Argyll Robertson pupils). Cerebral and spinal cord (anterior spinal artery) vessels may be affected. Epilepsy, confusion, aphasia, monoplegia, hemiplegia, or paraplegia, are just some of the ways in which late meningovascular syphilis can present.

Parenchymatous neurosyphilis may present as general paralysis of the insane, tabes dorsalis, or, rarely, a combination of the two. General paralysis of the insane is the result of a chronic progressive meningoencephalitis with resulting cerebral atrophy 10–20 years after the original primary infection. Manifestations of the disease are a poor memory, lack of judgment and insight, delusions, confusion and mood swings, and sometimes convulsions. The signs can include a fine tremor of the lips, tongue, and hands; dysarthria; occasionally Argyll Robertson pupils and optic atrophy; hyperactive tendon reflexes; and extensor plantar responses (due to lesions of the pyramidal tract). Late in the disease the patient may suffer from dementia, a spastic paraplegia, and urinary and faecal incontinence.

Tabes dorsalis is characterised by increasing ataxia, failing vision, sphincter disturbances, and attacks of severe pains. These pains are described as "lightening" since they occur as acute stabbing pain commonly in the legs. Attacks are fleeting or last a few days and classically occur at right angles to the limb. Paraesthesiae, incontinence, impotence, and tabetic crises may occur. These crises usually occur acutely and affect the stomach, rectum, bladder, urethra, kidneys, and larynx. The gastric crisis is the most common and the symptoms of epigastric pain and vomiting can be mistaken for an acute surgical abdomen.

General paralysis of the insane

Symptoms

Early	Late
Irritability	Defective judgement
Fatigability	Lack of insight
Inefficiency	Depression or euphoria
Personality changes	Confusion and disorientation
Headaches	Delusions
Impaired memory	Seizures
Tremors	Transient paralysis and aphasia

Signs

Expressionless facies
Tremor of lips, tongue, and hands
Dysarthria
Impairment of handwriting
Hyperactive tendon reflexes
Pupillary abnormalities
Optic atrophy
Convulsions
Extensor plantar responses

Syphilis: clinical features

Tabes dorsalis	
Symptoms	*Signs*
Lightning pains	Argyll Robertson pupils
Ataxia	Absent ankle reflexes
Bladder disturbance	Absent knee reflexes
Paraesthesiae	Absent biceps and triceps reflexes
Tabetic crises	Romberg's sign
Visual loss	Impaired vibration sense
Rectal incontinence	Impaired position sense
Deafness	Impaired sense of touch and pain
Impotence	Optic atrophy
	Ocular palsies
	Charcot's joints

The signs of tabes dorsalis are largely due to degeneration of the posterior columns: absent ankle and knee reflexes (rarely biceps and triceps), impaired vibration and position sense, and a positive Romberg's sign. Argyll Robertson pupils are found in half of the cases and optic atrophy in a fifth. Charcot's arthropathy is rare, found in fewer than 10% of cases. The joints (knee, hip, ankle, spine, feet) are grossly disorganised and hypermobile with osteophyte formation and loose bodies in the joint. Finally, perforating ulcers of the feet can be found.

Cardiovascular syphilis

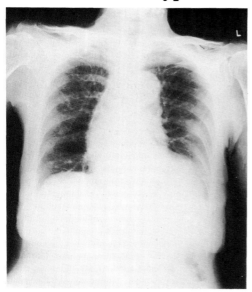

Cardiovascular syphilis most commonly occurs in large vessels, but medium and small sized ones may also be affected. The aorta is affected by an aortitis (with or without coronary ostial stenosis), an aneurysm of the ascending part, and aortic incompetence. Aneurysms of innominate, carotid, and subclavian vessels have also been described. Early changes are symptomless. Advancing aortitis may result in dull substernal pain or angina whereas aortic incompetence can present with acute left ventricular failure, paroxysmal nocturnal dyspnoea, and angina. The symptoms of aortic aneurysm vary depending on site; if in the ascending part (the commonest site) there may be dull substernal pain or angina and left ventricular failure. The symptoms of an aneurysm affecting the arch usually result from the pressure on structures within the superior mediastinum. Thus, stridor and cough (trachea), dysphagia (oesophagus), breathlessness (left bronchus), hoarseness (left recurrent laryngeal nerve), and Horner's syndrome (sympathetic chain) may occur. Finally, pressure on the superior vena cava can result in congested veins in the head and neck and cyanosis. The signs of cardiovascular disease are no different from those of aortic incompetence and aneurysms from other causes.

Gummatous syphilis

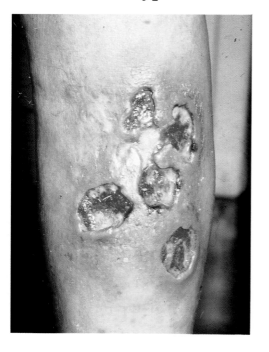

Gummas are granulamatous lesions appearing three to 12 years after the primary infection. Gummas may occur on the skin or mucous membranes and in bone or viscera. Skin lesions are usually nodular. They can occur anywhere on the skin and appear as small groups of painless lesions which are indolent, firm, coppery red, and about 0·5–1 cm in diameter. If subcutaneous tissue is affected the lesions start as smooth hard swellings which eventually break down into well circumscribed punched out ulcers which, when they heal, leave typical tissue paper scarring. These occur on the leg, face, and scalp. Lesions in mucous membrane appear as punched out ulcers on the hard and soft palate, uvula, tongue, larynx, pharynx, and nasal septum. Bone and visceral gummas are extremely rare, affecting the tibia, skull, clavicle, sternum, and femur, liver, brain, oesophagus, stomach, lung, and testes.

SYPHILIS: DIAGNOSIS AND MANAGEMENT

History
Physical examination
±
Dark ground microscopy
Serology
Lumbar puncture
Chest radiography and screening

Establishing a diagnosis of syphilis, whatever the stage of the disease, can be difficult and it is wise for all suspected cases to be referred for specialised tests and management in a department of genitourinary medicine. The diagnosis can be confirmed by the history, physical examination, and one or all of four tests—dark ground microscopy, serology, examination of cerebrospinal fluid, and radiology. Which of these tests appear as positive will depend on the clinical stage of the patient's syphilis.

Dark ground microscopy

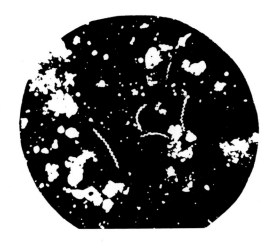

Dark ground microscopy can be used to establish the diagnosis from the lesions of primary and secondary syphilis or occasionally from material obtained by puncture of inguinal nodes (after recent topical application of antiseptic or antibiotic or when lesions are healed or concealed). The presence of oral commensal treponemes makes microscopy unreliable for mouth lesions. Three separate specimens from the lesion(s) should be examined by dark ground microscopy initially and, if necessary, on three consecutive days. This is done by cleaning the lesion with a gauze swab soaked in normal saline and squeezing it to encourage a serum exudate. The serum is then scraped off the lesion and placed on the three slides. After a cover slip has been placed on the material microscopy can be performed. Dark ground microscopy is a vital test since in primary syphilis it may be the only positive means of establishing the diagnosis. Considerable experience is required to recognise *Treponema pallidum*. It is bluish white, closely coiled (8–24), and 6–20 µm long. There are three characteristic movements of the treponeme: watch spring, corkscrew, and angular. Serological tests for syphilis are not always positive when primary lesions occur; the tests do not give positive results until about two weeks after the appearance of the chancre, about three to five weeks after infection.

Serological tests

Non-specific tests

Venereal Disease Research Laboratory test

Rapid plasma reagin test

Wasermann reaction

Specific tests

Absorbed fluorescent treponemal antibody test

Treponema pallidum haemagglutination test

Biological false positive reactions
Acute — Chronic
Infections | After immunisation | Autoimmune disease | Leprosy

The serological tests used in the diagnosis of syphilis are either non-specific or specific.

Non-specific tests—The most useful non-specific tests are either the Venereal Disease Research Laboratory test (VDRL) or the rapid plasma reagin (RPR) test which have now replaced the Wassermann reaction. Essentially these tests depend on the appearance of antibody (reagin) in the serum, and this may not occur until three to five weeks after the patient has contracted the infection. Thus the VDRL/RPR tests will give positive results in only about 75% of cases of primary syphilis. They are quantitative tests and this can be useful in assessing the stage and activity of the disease. The VDRL test is a flocculation test. Positive results may occur for three reasons. Firstly, technical errors may occur because of mistakes in collection, labelling, and reporting of specimens or the use of faulty materials. The moral is that the diagnosis of syphilis should never be made on the basis of only one set of tests. Secondly, positive results occur in syphilis and other treponemal conditions similar to syphilis (yaws, bejel, and pinta), but in such instances the specific tests will also be positive. Thirdly, there may be acute or chronic biological false positive reactions.

Syphilis: diagnosis and management

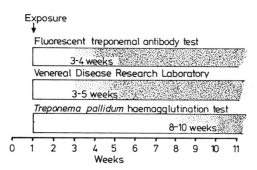

	Stage of disease			
	Primary %	Secondary %	Latent %	Late %
Veneral Disease Research Laboratory test	75	100	75	75
Treponema pallidum haemagglutination test	60	100	97	100
Fluorescent treponemal antibody test	90	100	97	100

Results positive	Diagnosis
None	Syphilis not present or very early primary syphilis
All	Untreated, recently treated, or latent syphilis
VDRL and FTA	Primary syphilis
TPHA and FTA	Treated syphilis or untreated latent or late
FTA only	Early primary syphilis—untreated or recently treated early syphilis
TPHA only	Treated syphilis
VDRL only	False positive reaction

Biological false positive reactions—The acute type of reaction is transient, lasting a few weeks to six months. Such reactions occur after viral infections (such as glandular fever, measles, chicken pox, mumps, herpes simplex and zoster, viral pneumonia) or after immunisation against typhoid and yellow fever. The chronic false positive reaction can last for many years or even a lifetime. It is seen particularly in autoimmune diseases (disseminated lupus erythematosis, haemolytic anaemia, thyroiditis) and rheumatoid arthritis. Sometimes the VDRL test is positive years before the patient develops one of these conditions. Specific tests for syphilis will be negative.

Specific tests—The two specific tests most often used to establish a diagnosis of treponemal disease are the absorbed fluorescent treponemal antibody test (FTA-ABS) and the *Treponema pallidum* haemagglutination (TPHA) test. The fluorescent treponemal antibody test is the first serological test (either specific or non-specific) to become positive; this usually occurs three to four weeks after infection. Thus this test is positive in 85–90% of cases of primary syphilis. In early untreated primary disease it may be the only positive serological test. (The FTA is not a routine screening test, therefore if early syphilis is suspected this test will need to be requested of the laboratory). It must not be forgotten, however, that all serological tests may be negative despite the presence of a primary lesion. The *Treponema pallidum* haemagglutination test is the last of the serological tests to become positive. Thus it will always be positive in the secondary stages of disease but only so in 60% of patients presenting with primary syphilis. As already emphasised, these specific tests can distinguish only between treponemal and non-treponemal disease but not between the different treponemal conditions. Occasionally a clinical distinction can be made, for example, between syphilis and yaws.

The findings of positive serological tests for syphilis should not necessarily be interpreted as showing that the patient has active or untreated latent disease. Thus, for example, in patients who have received adequate treatment the VDRL test may still be positive (particularly if treated late on in the infection). Responses to the fluorescent treponemal antibody and *Treponema pallidum* haemagglutination tests often remain positive for life despite adequate treatment.

Syphilis has been controlled in the United Kingdom largely because of the policy of screening patients attending antenatal clinics, departments of genitourinary medicine, and blood transfusion centres and by selective use in neurological and psychiatric assessment of certain patients. Currently the best combination of tests for screening for treponemal disease is the VDRL test and the *Treponema pallidum* haemagglutination test.

Cerebrospinal fluid and radiology

Investigations of cerebrospinal fluid
● Cell count
● Total protein
● IgG estimation (or Lange colloidal gold curve)
● Venereal Disease Research Laboratory, *Treponema pallidum* haemagglutination, and fluorescent treponemal antibody tests

Abnormalities of the cerebrospinal fluid may be found at any stage of syphilis and may occur early (primary and secondary stages) without symptoms. Many clinicians therefore examine the cerebrospinal fluid a year after treatment of early disease before discharging the patients as cured. Lumbar puncture may also be necessary to exclude neurosyphilis or as part of the investigation of any patient with suspected latent disease. The following tests can be performed on cerebrospinal fluid: cell count, total protein, IgG estimation, or Lange colloidal gold curve (no longer used widely), and the three serological tests. The findings vary according to the type of neurosyphilis. A cell count above 0.005×10^9 lymphocytes per litre and protein above 40 g/l would be considered abnormal. The VDRL test on the fluid is unreliable in diagnosing neurosyphilis since it is negative in up to half of all patients with active neurosyphilis. A positive fluorescent treponemal antibody or *Treponema pallidum* haemagglutination test result, or both, can result from a transudate of

IgG specific for *Treponema pallidum* in patients whose disease has been adequately treated. It therefore, does not indicate active disease of the nervous system; negative results, however, virtually rule out neurosyphilis.

The final diagnostic procedure in the assessment of a patient with latent disease or cardiovascular disease is a chest radiograph (posteroanterior, left oblique) to show the arch of the aorta and screening to detect aortic dilatation. More specialised tests such as catheterisation may subsequently be indicated.

Treatment and prognosis

Herxheimer reaction		
		% Of patients affected
Primary		50%
Secondary		70-90%
Early latent		25%
Late latent		20%
Neurosyphilis	general paralysis	50-75%
	tabes	Rare
Cardiovascular		Rare

Changes in cerebrospinal fluid in neurosyphilis

		Stage of disease			
	Asymptomatic	Meningovascular		Parenchymatous	
		Early	Late	General paralysis of the insane	Tabes dorsalis
Cell count	±	+++	++	++	+
Protein	+	++	++	++	+
FTA	+	+	+	+	+/−
VDRL	−	+	±	++	+/−
TPHA	+	+	+	+	+/−
Pressure	Normal	++	±	Normal	Normal

Penicillin remains the cornerstone of the treatment of all types of syphilis. In primary and secondary syphilis aqueous procaine penicillin should be given for 10 days. Successful treatment depends on obtaining a minimum serum concentration of 30 IU/l and maintaining this over a long period. If there is any anxiety about patients returning or if they cannot attend daily, erythromycin or tetracycline (except for neurosyphilis) can be substituted. Also these can be used in patients allergic to penicillin. Since the cure rate is lower with these, many physicians will repeat treatment after three months.

The Jarisch–Herxheimer reaction is common in primary and secondary syphilis and patients must be warned that fever and flu-like symptoms may occur 3–12 hours after the first injection; occasionally the chancre or skin lesions enlarge or become more widespread. Aspirin is recommended.

Other stages or manifestations of syphilis are also treated with procaine penicillin. Steroids, to eliminate the Herxheimer reaction, are used only in patients with neurosyphilis or cardiovascular syphilis who may develop focal lesions (cerebrovascular or coronary artery occlusion) and mania, confusion, and psychosis.

The prognosis of treated syphilis depends on the stage of the disease and degree of tissue damage in the cardiovascular and neurological systems. Thus adequate treatment of primary, secondary, and latent stages and asymptomatic neurosyphilis will result in cure and halt progression of the disease. The prognosis in symptomatic cardiovascular and neurosyphilis is variable. In general the inflammatory process is arrested by adequate treatment but the tissue damage may be too great to prevent an improvement in symptoms.

Contact tracing must be carried out on all sexual contacts that a patient with early infectious syphilis has had in the preceding three to six months. In late syphilis, when the patient is no longer infectious, serological testing is probably only practicable in the patient's regular partner. If late syphilis is diagnosed in a mother it may be necessary to test her children. Syphilis during pregnancy is discussed in the next chapter. Syphilis is a complex disease and its diagnosis, management, and follow up should not be undertaken by the non-specialist.

Syphilis: diagnosis and management

Treatment of syphilis

Stage	Standard treatment	Alternatives		Prognosis
Primary and secondary	Aqueous procaine penicillin 600 000 units/day 10 days →	If penicillin allergy: Erythromycin } 500 mg four times Oxytetracycline } a day 30 days		Excellent Relapse exceptionally first year
Latent: early (≤2 years duration)	Aqueous procaine penicillin 600 000 units/day 10 days ↗	If patient unable to attend daily: Benzathine penicillin 2·4 MU once only		
late (>2 years)	Aqueous procaine penicillin 900 000 units/day 21 days →	If penicillin allergy or unable to attend daily: Erythromycin } 500 mg four times Oxytetracycline } a day 30 days		Excellent
Neurosyphilis and cardiovascular syphilis	Aqueous procaine penicillin 900 000 units/day 21 days + prednisone 5 mg four times daily for one day before penicillin, and then same dose for two days after	If penicillin allergy: Oxytetracycline 500 mg four times a day 30 days Doxycycline 200 mg once a day 30 days	} Not suitable for neurosyphilis	Depends on type of neurosyphilis and extent of cardiovascular disease
Gummatous	Aqueous procaine penicillin 600 000 units/day 15 days	If penicillin allergy: Erythromycin } 500 mg four times Tetracycline } a day for 15 days		

PREGNANCY AND THE NEONATE

Herpes	Syphilis
Chlamydia	Cytomegalovirus
Gonorrhoea	

The consequences of sexually transmitted diseases for the unborn or newly born child are extremely emotive, when they need not be so. Most of the material diseases that can affect the fetus or neonate can be prevented or are usually not serious if recognised and treated early. The unpreventable or unprevented diseases, however, although rare, may have serious and lifelong consequences.

Genital herpes

Risk of neonatal herpes

Primary attack in mother at delivery 50%

Recurrent attack in mother at delivery 5%

There are two problems associated with infection with genital herpes simplex virus during pregnancy: congenital infection and neonatal infection. It is theoretically possible for transplacental transmission to occur but evidence for this is poor. If it does occur it is likely to result in fetal death and spontaneous abortion. The reported annual incidence of neonatal herpes is low in the United Kingdom (about 2/100 000 live births, 14 cases) and higher in the USA (ranging from 1/3000 to 1/20 000 live births, 180–1190 cases) Neonatal infection can occur if the mother has active herpes at the time of delivery, either with lesions or without (asymptomatic viral shedding). The risk to the neonate is greater from primary than from recurrent episodes in the mother.

Up to 60% of babies with neonatal herpes are born to mothers with no symptoms or signs of the disease at the time of delivery. These women may be shedding virus asymptomatically, or the infant may acquire the infection after delivery from maternal labial herpes or herpes infection in one of the medical or nursing staff or other babies.

Sources of neonatal herpes infection

- Mother–labial, cervical, vulval lesions

- Medical and nursing staff, other babies

Neonatal herpes can be fatal within the first few weeks or result in permanent brain damage in the survivors. The disease can present either in a localised or disseminated form. The overall mortality is about 60%.

Management

The high risk of infection to the neonate and high fatality rate make the correct management of genital herpes in pregnancy important. A correct and substantiated diagnosis must be made as early as possible, and the patient must be clearly informed about how her pregnancy will be managed.

Despite the high mortality, neonatal herpes is rare and there is no need to screen all pregnant women for the condition. The traditional approach has been to suggest that monitoring during pregnancy should be limited to women who give a history of herpes or who develop it during pregnancy. Thus, from 36 weeks onwards weekly viral cultures could be taken from the cervix and vulva regardless of whether lesions are present or not. Caesarean section would be carried out only if active lesions—recurrent or primary—or viral shedding without lesions is found at 39–40 weeks. If the mother goes into spontaneous labour before the elective procedure is performed caesarean section could still be indicated up to four hours after rupture of the membranes. This view is now questioned on the basis of cost (in the USA it is calculated that the cost of avoiding one case of neonatal herpes through screening during late pregnancy is about

	Incidence (%)	Mortality (%)
Localised		
Central nervous system meningoencephalitis	35	50-75
Eye conjunctivitis, keratitis, chorioretinitis	15	0
Skin vesicular lesions	50	10
Oral cavity vesicular lesions	50	0
Disseminated		
Multiple organs affected, including brain, lung, stomach, kidneys, adrenals, spleen, liver, heart, bone marrow, etc	35-50	85
Overall mortality		60%

$1·8m) and low risk to the neonate if the mother only has recurrent herpes. It is suggested therefore that only those women who have clinical lesions at the time of delivery should be recommended for caesarean section. Until further studies are performed, however, it is difficult to indicate the correct up to date strategy.

Despite this monitoring, a few babies with neonatal herpes will still be born. Trials with vidarabine and acyclovir have both been shown to be effective in the treatment of such neonates. The problem with both drugs, particularly on those babies who have herpes encephalitis, is that they improve survival but many of the survivors have severe neurological impairment.

Chlamydial infections

Conjunctivitis	Pneumonia
Otitis media	Failure to thrive
Nasopharyngitis	

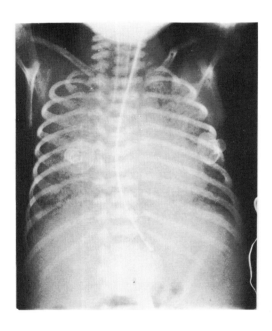

Chlamydia trachomatis can be transmitted by direct inoculation into the neonate's eye or by inhalation of infected material during birth; 30–50% of infants born to infected mothers will develop eye disease and 10–20% a pneumonia. The eye disease appears one to three weeks after birth and varies from a mild inclusion conjunctivitis to a purulent and severe ophthalmia with oedema of the eyelids and palpebral conjunctiva. In half of all cases the condition is bilateral. If untreated the condition usually resolves spontaneously, but in rare instances it can progress to conjunctival scarring and micropannus formation.

A nasopharyngitis or pneumonia, resulting from the inhalation of infected material at birth, usually presents one to three months after birth. The infant with pneumonia is usually afebrile with a paroxysmal staccato cough, tachypnoea, occasionally apnoea, and sometimes an associated nasal discharge and otitis media. There is failure to thrive in most cases. The chest radiograph shows hyperexpansion with bilateral symmetrical diffuse interstitial and patchy alveolar infiltrates. About half the infants also have conjunctivitis or a history of it.

Diagnosis—Eye, nasopharyngeal, or lung disease due to chlamydia is diagnosed by isolating the organism. The pneumonia is usually associated with eosinophilia, raised serum IgG and IgM concentrations, and raised titres to *C trachomatis*.

Treatment—Chlamydial conjunctivitis should be treated systemically since up to half the infants may later develop a nasopharyngitis or pneumonia. Application of ointment into the eye is difficult and unnecessary. Saline bathing can be used. Erythromycin ethylsuccinate should be used in divided doses up to a total of 50 mg/kg body weight/day for 14–21 days. The pneumonia should be treated with the same regimen.

Both the mother and father should be examined to look for *C trachomatis* and any other concurrent sexually acquired condition.

Gonococcal infections

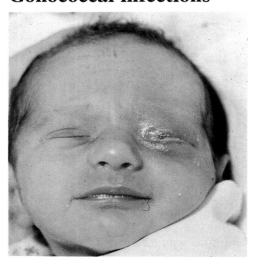

Gonococcal conjunctivitis is transmitted in the same way as chlamydial infection. The inflammation and purulent discharge are usually evident within a few days of birth. Rarely colonisation of the pharynx and rectum and a gonococcal septicaemia (similar to that found in adults) can be seen.

Diagnosis is by microscopy and culture of infected material from the eye. Systemic treatment is required. As with chlamydial ophthalmia local insertion of antibiotic into the eye is not sufficient or necessary but saline bathing may be applied. Systemic penicillin is required—for example, benzylpenicillin 50 000 units/kg body weight daily in divided doses. It is preferable to give this in two doses a day for three days. The mother and her sexual contacts will also require investigation and, if necessary, treatment.

Ophthalmia neonatorum (a conjunctivitis within 21 days of birth) is notifiable. A chlamydial or gonococcal infection should always be suspected in an infant with a sticky eye, and these two organisms should be excluded in every case. These conditions are not the commonest causes of a sticky eye in neonates but the increasing incidence of chlamydial infections now makes this form of ophthalmia five times more common than gonococcal.

Syphilis

Treatment of mother with syphilis during pregnancy	
Early infectious syphilis	Procaine penicillin 600 000 units intramuscularly daily for 10 days
Other stages	Same as in non-pregnant state
If allergic to penicillin	Erythromycin

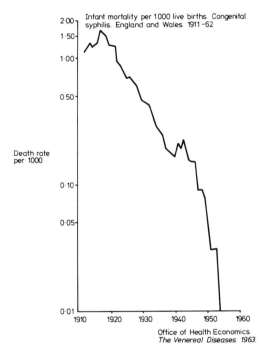

Infant mortality per 1000 live births. Congenital syphilis. England and Wales 1911-62

Death rate per 1000

Office of Health Economics
The Venereal Diseases 1963.

Clinical features of congenital syphilis	
Early	Similar to adult secondary disease: rash, mucous membrane lesions, lymphadenopathy, ± lesions of bone, viscera, eye, central nervous system
Latent (early and late)	No clinical signs of active disease ± stigmata Positive serological test results
Late (⩾2)	Similar to adult late disease Interstitial keratitis, osteoperiostitis, joint effusions, usually knees (Clutton's joints) Gumma hard and soft palate, pharynx 8th Nerve deafness Neurological features Cardiovascular complications Stigmata

Unlike infections with herpes, chlamydia, and gonorrhoea, which are acquired at birth, syphilis is a prenatal infection. Fetal infection may occur at any time during pregnancy. It is more likely to occur if the mother has primary, secondary, or early latent syphilis since considerable numbers of organisms are present in the circulation during these stages. The infectivity when the mother has untreated primary or secondary disease is virtually 100%. This decreases the longer the mother has been suffering from her disease. It is uncommon for a woman with late syphilis to give birth to a child with congenital disease but it is possible, even though previous pregnancies may have been normal.

Congenital syphilis is no longer a public health problem in developed countries. Latest figures show only nine cases per year in children aged under 2 years in the United Kingdom and no deaths. The low incidence of congenital syphilis in the United Kingdom is due largely to the control of early acquired infectious syphilis in women and through screening all pregnant women for syphilis. Serological tests should be carried out at the first antenatal visit. It is still possible for the mother to become infected after this or for her to be incubating the disease with negative serological results. Women at high risk of infection should therefore have the tests repeated in the final trimester.

A pregnant woman found to have syphilis is likely to be suffering from early infectious syphilis. If so the appropriate treatment is aqueous procaine penicillin 600 000 units intramuscularly daily for 10 days. Other stages of syphilis require the same treatment as used in the non-pregnant patient (see previous chapter). Penicillin given during pregnancy produces a prevention and cure rate of virtually 100%. If the mother is allergic to penicillin, erythromycin (not the estolate) should be used at a level of 500 mg six hourly for 15 days or for 30 days if she has latent infection. Placental transfer of this drug can be inadequate so it is essential to be absolutely certain that the patient has a genuine sensitivity to penicillin. If penicillin cannot be used for the mother the baby should have a course of penicillin at birth as a precaution.

Even if the mother has had an adequate course of penicillin during pregnancy the baby should be examined and serological tests carried out. Despite treatment of the mother, her serological results may still be positive at term. As passive transfer of antibody from the mother to the baby can occur, time must be allowed for this carryover to disappear (at least six weeks). Thus tests are carried out on the baby at six weeks and three months after birth.

There is some debate whether treatment in subsequent pregnancies is indicated. Some clinicians believe that this is desirable because of the possible persistence of the treponeme in the body after treatment and subsequent transplacental transfer. If the mother has been followed up for two years after treatment and discharged as cured an alternative approach is not to treat her in subsequent pregnancies but to perform serological tests for syphilis on the baby at the age of 3 months.

Congenital syphilis

When it occurs, congenital syphilis is classified into early, latent, and late stages. The clinical picture varies depending on the stage. The lesions of late syphilis can appear at varying intervals during the child's life.

The lesions of early and late congenital syphilis may heal but leave

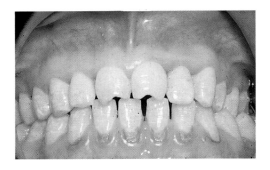

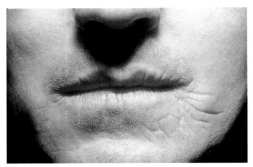

stigmata. On the *face and mouth* a saddle nose deformity and collapse of the bridge of the nose may occur as a result of rhinitis and gumma of the nasal septum. The face may look flat owing to impaired development of maxillae, and frontal bossing (Parrot's nodes) can be seen. Linear scars (rhagades) around the angles of the mouth result from healed mucocutaneous lesions of early disease. In the *teeth* the upper central incisors are smaller than normal and peg or barrel shaped and have a classically notched centre (Hutchinson's incisors). The molars can also be affected and show a rounded appearance (Moon's molars). In the *eyes* scarring can remain as a result of earlier choroidal involvement and opacities of the cornea and ghost vessels can be seen as a result of interstitial keratitis. *Bone lesions* include sabre tibia following previous osteoperiostitis.

Early congenital syphilis—The clinical picture may arouse suspicion, but confirmatory tests are required. Clinical manifestations may present only after several weeks. Dark field microscopy from skin lesions or nasal discharge can establish the diagnosis immediately. Positive serological findings are confirmatory. Serological tests for syphilis (Venereal Diseases Research Laboratory and *Treponema pallidum* haemagglutination tests) should be performed at birth, but passive transfer from the mother will make interpretation of these impossible early on, and they should be repeated at 6 and 12 weeks. A rising titre is compatible with congenital disease. In the last few years the fluorescent treponemal antibody absorbed IgM test has been used in an attempt to differentiate passive transfer from true congenital disease at an early stage. Specific IgM in the neonate has been thought to indicate congenital disease; unfortunately false positive and negative results do occur and it is probably not wise to rely on this test for such an important diagnosis. In the presence of positive results to standard serological tests (Venereal Diseases Research Laboratory and *Treponema pallidum* haemagglutination tests) there is no substitute for waiting a number of weeks. The baby will not suffer from delay in treatment, but the parents may, of course, be anxious. Their anxiety has to be weighed against making an early diagnosis that may be wrong, and labelling the baby with the diagnosis of congenital syphilis for the rest of its life, making the parents guilty about the disease that they have passed on.

Latent and late congenital syphilis—Most cases of latent and late syphilis are identified because of incidental serological tests for syphilis. Sometimes cases are found when the patient or parent consults because of impairment of hearing (nerve deafness) or sight, swollen knee (Clutton's joints), or because other gross stigmata of disease are present. Serological tests will invariably give positive results. Other features, such as old interstitial keratitis and ghost vessels, should be looked for by slit lamp examination.

Early and late congenital syphilis—The treatment in early congenital syphilis is intramuscular benzylpenicillin or procaine penicillin 50 000 units/kg body weight for 10 days. In late congenital syphilis the treatment is as for the equivalent stage in late acquired adult syphilis. The daily dose for children or adolescents is adjusted according to weight.

PSYCHOLOGICAL AND SEXUAL PROBLEMS

DAVID GOLDMEIER

Psychological factors are major influences determining whether or not sexual intercourse will take place. Once sexually transmitted disease is acquired, or its presence is feared, the patient's emotions are difficult to dismiss.

Unless a patient has been raped, acquisition of sexually transmitted disease can be seen as the result of a more or less conscious decision taken before physical contact. Various factors influence patients in deciding whether or not intercourse should take place.

Most patients who attend sexually transmitted disease clinics will talk relatively freely about sexual matters. With gentle coaxing they will also discuss their psychological problems.

HIV disease apart, psychological illness is obvious in 1–2% of attenders at sexually transmitted disease clinics and is detectable by validated questionnaire in up to 40% of patients.

Psychological and psychosexual problems encountered in a clinic may be classified into:
a. Primary psychiatric disease states,
b. Psychiatric disease secondary to sexually transmitted disease, or
c. Sexual, marital, and relationship problems.

Psychosocial factors influencing whether sexual intercourse takes place or not

Factors	Explanation
Age	Libido decreases with age
Religion	Many religions have ethos of monogamy or celibacy and do not accept extramarital intercourse
Ethnic or cultural	Wife sharing in some cultures
Prostitution	Sexual contact certain unless prostitute discriminates against "high risk" client
Illicit drugs or alcohol	May cause disinhibition
Personality	Extroverts more likely to have casual intercourse
Sexual orientation	Before AIDS homosexual men had high rate of partner change
"Infatuation"	"Falling in love" likely to lead to intercourse (biological? cultural?)
Unusual environment	Holidays or conferences—casual intercourse more likely
Psychiatric illness	Depression—decreased chance of intercourse
Hypomania—increased chance of intercourse

Primary psychiatric disease states

Classification of hypochondriasis

Psychiatric phenomenon	Description of phenomenon	Psychiatric illness underlying phenomenon
Phobia	Fear of disease dispelled by discussion with doctor, but returns quickly	Anxiety, neurotic depression
Delusion	Fixed false conviction of disease not altered by discussion	Monosymptomatic delusion, schizophrenia, psychotic depression

Most patients attending a sexually transmitted disease clinic worry about having such an infection. Doctors must reassure patients in clear, simple language. If two sessions, say 10–15 minutes each, have not achieved this result, and the patient still believes he or she has a sexually transmitted disease, the patient may be said to have hypochondriasis. Hypochondriasis can be further classified into phobias and delusions.

Phobias are best managed by cognitive behaviour therapy and tricyclic antidepressants used as anxiolytics. Delusions should be managed by the psychiatrists.

Psychological and sexual problems
Psychiatric disease secondary to STD

Gonococcal and non-gonococcal urethritis

Both of these conditions are usually easily and rapidly treated, and early intercourse after tests of cure in an otherwise stable relationship may help to heal the psychological wounds that one or both partners may feel. Unfortunately non-gonococcal urethritis may be recurrent or even chronic, and the man may have been told not to resume intercourse until inflammation has subsided. Prolonged sexual abstinence puts a profound strain on the relationship, which is exacerbated if the woman is (incorrectly) told to attend for treatment at each recurrence. There is a lot to be said for seeing the couple together, so that their treatment can be coordinated. The physician can then also gauge the effects of and the necessity for sexual abstinence, can assess their relationship, and can facilitate discussion about the urethritis and underlying problems in the relationship.

Prostatic pain

Patients with prostatadynia and prostatitis are commonly anxious and some are depressed. Reassurance, antidepressants, and hypnotherapy can all lower the pain threshold.

Pelvic pain

Pelvic pain may be caused by pelvic inflammatory disease or by other disease within the pelvis. Many patients with pelvic inflammatory disease complain of deep dyspareunia and are also either infertile or subfertile. As well as dealing with the feelings of loss of health and fertility, the doctor may usefully see the individual or couple to pinpoint problems that have arisen out of one or both partners having had intercourse with others and to discuss the resulting feelings of anger and resentment.

Genital herpes

Primary genital herpes is distressing not only because of the physical symptoms but also because of the grief reaction that can follow the realisation of a future with a chronic, painful, sometimes frequently recurring genital infection that can be passed on to the very people the patient wants to cherish and protect. The patient may have heard jokes about herpes, have heard friends equating herpes with AIDS, and may have sensed that friends or even prospective sexual partners have a negative attitude to herpes. All of this may result in a tarnished self image or even worse in a total loss of self esteem.

There is an association between the degree of non-psychotic psychiatric illness, assessed at the time of the first attack, and the time to the first recurrence—that is, the greater the degree of psychiatric illness the sooner the first recurrence. Patients with frequent recurrence of genital herpes (every four weeks or more often) need to be given time to discuss their feelings and their herpes. Commonly found factors that tend to increase the rate of recurrence are lack of sleep, adverse life circumstances,

and often the presence of the infection itself (which precludes a satisfactory sexual relationship). Open, frank, and sympathetic discussion within specially designated clinics is very likely to beneficially alter the patient's self image and may even prevent the recurrences that so depress many patients.

It is surprising how commonly patients continue to adhere to false ideas about genital herpes. The possibility of developing cervical cancer, being infertile, causing fatal infections in their babies, and never having another intimate relationship because all prospective sexual partners will be frightened away are some of these exaggerated fears.

Genital candidiasis

Frequent recurrences of genital candidiasis may leave both partners confused, frustrated, and angry about the supposed source of the problem. A steady, stable relationship should be able to withstand this problem with a minimum of counselling to the woman. The finding of *Candida albicans* in genital secretions may tempt the physician to make an organic diagnosis, whereas the real problem may be vaginismus along with the incidental discovery of *Candida albicans*.

Trichomoniasis and anaerobic vaginosis

These conditions usually cause an offensive vaginal discharge, which both partners can find offputting. After treatment, in spite of the absence of any objective odour, the woman may have lost confidence in her physiological body odour, and the man may mistake the normal musty vaginal odour for the previous abnormal smell. The couple may need to be seen together, to hear the physician assure them of the normality of the discharge.

Syphilis

Syphilis is a special case, whether congenital or acquired. Many older patients still think of syphilis as "worse than cancer," and a few may have catastrophic reactions when they find out the nature of their illness. Congenital syphilis presenting in later life may devastate the patient when he realises the implication of his disease in respect of his parents.

HIV disease

To a greater or lesser extent all patients with HIV disease have psychological problems. The major patient groups at risk in Britain often have psychological problems before becoming infected. Homosexual men may become anxious or depressed because of actual or feared non-acceptance of their sexuality by family, friends, or employers. Intravenous drug abusers have the multitude of problems that their addiction brings, apart from the personality disorders that antedate the drug abuse.

All patients should be counselled before an HIV antibody test is undertaken, as important issues may need to be discussed.

Important issues discussed in counselling before patients tested for antibody to HIV

(1) General facts about HIV disease
(2) Meaning of positive test result
(3) Meaning of negative test result
(4) Confidentiality of the result
(5) Handling stress in relation to taking the test
(6) Social difficulties that may be encountered if result is positive

Social rejection by hostile family and friends and dismissal by employers and insurance companies must be considered. Counselling may evoke very uncomfortable feelings, particularly when the patient has never really considered a positive result. Nowadays, however, most patients decide at the first visit to have the test, having given the test some thought before they even come to the clinic. In a minority of patients it may be best to postpone the test. For instance, in the case of a physically well homosexual man whose partner died of AIDS six months previously, and who is now depressed and abuses alcohol daily because of fear of HIV disease,

the correct initial steps are to withdraw him from alcohol, give antidepressants and psychotherapy when necessary, and to return to the issue of HIV disease when his mental state has improved.

In spite of pretest counselling, about a third of all patients who are told of their HIV positivity have a shortlived adjustment (grief) reaction. Half of these will develop a more protracted reaction lasting weeks or months, suffering some or all of the symptoms of anxiety, depression, hypochodriasis, fatigue, and lethargy. As the latter symptoms overlap with those of advanced HIV disease, careful physical and psychological assessment is mandatory.

It is now generally accepted that HIV subacute encephalopathy and its associated dementia are unlikely to develop in patients unless they have ARC or AIDS. Once the patient has ARC or AIDS, psychiatric symptoms should be considered to be organic (pulmonary, hepatic, and renal malfunction, cerebral infections, tumours, or dementia) until organic disease is excluded. Depression is commonly found in patients with AIDS. Loss of health and youthful looks, financial worries, and dying itself are but some of the issues that may underlie the depression. Most AIDS centres now have psychiatrists with a special interest in the management of these problems.

Sexual, marital, and relationship problems

It is important that the genitourinary physician should not force an "innocently" infected partner to accept his or her diagnosis when it is already implicitly understood. Sometimes it is better not to be explicit. Rather, the patient should be given room to manoeuvre by saying, for instance, "Is there anything more you would like to know?" Often the answer is "No." Relationships and marriages can be saved by careful and considered explanations.

The underaged and rape victims, irrespective of the patient's sex, are not uncommonly seen in sexually transmitted disease clinics to have screening tests. They always need careful, gentle, thorough, and sympathetic examination and explanation, and may need long term

counselling if they are not having it elsewhere. When child abuse is considered to be a possibility, paediatricians and the hospital social workers should be consulted.

A number of sexually transmitted disease clinics now offer facilities for managing psychosexual (erectile dysfunction, premature ejaculation, vaginismus, orgasmic dysfunction) and marital problems that are unrelated to sexually transmitted disease. Many of the patients are self referred, perhaps seeking the anonymity and confidentiality that sexually transmitted disease clinics afford. There may be organic causes for erectile failure and these should be considered before embarking on psychosexual therapies.

METHODS OF CONTROL

The sexually transmitted diseases represent one of the major health problems in the world today. The size of the problem in the United Kingdom has been referred to earlier (see first chapter), and the position in the rest of the world is no less serious. About 200 000 000 new cases of gonorrhoea and 40 000 000 new cases of syphilis are notified throughout the world each year; these are undoubtedly underestimates. The demographic, sociological, and behavioural changes seen throughout the world in the past 30 years will continue to contribute towards an even greater problem in controlling sexually acquired infections in the future. The advent of human immunodeficiency virus (HIV) infection and AIDS has highlighted the importance of good control programmes for the sexually transmitted diseases. In general those countries with an efficient service for these diseases have found it easier to control the HIV–AIDS epidemic.

Early diagnosis and treatment are cheap; late sequelae of untreated disease are expensive. For example, if a good control programme exists most cases of pelvic inflammatory disease are preventable; if not prevented, however, the psychological, social, and monetary costs are large. Such costs increase further with developments in medical technology; thus, fallopian tube microsurgery and in vitro fertilisation and implantation of human embryos can now be performed at great expense in those sterilised by pelvic inflammatory disease. Prevention is better than cure, which is better than late intervention.

There are several complementary ways in which sexually transmitted diseases can be controlled. In the United Kingdom the most important way is through the provision of adequate diagnostic and treatment facilities in departments of genitourinary medicine. The aims of this service are to offer prompt diagnosis and treatment, minimise the incidence of complications, trace and treat the infected partners of patients, and educate patients, the public, and health care workers.

Methods of control

Facilities for diagnosis and treatment
Contact tracing
Education
Personal prophylaxis
Research

Aims of genitourinary medicine

- Prompt diagnosis and treatment
- Minimise incidence of complications and disability
- Trace and treat sexual contacts
- Education

Clinics

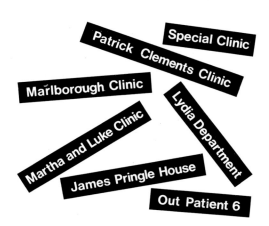

There are 230 departments of genitourinary medicine in the United Kingdom. Most clinics are situated within a general hospital, in the outpatient department or in their own purpose built premises. Unfortunately, some are still found in dingy basements or down dark alleyways. Facilities should alleviate, not create, stigma and be readily accessible for self referral. Some departments are called after physicians, apostles, or battles and others are termed "Special department" or given a number or letter. These differences make it difficult for patients to find their bearings and only add to their alienation, presenting a further hurdle to consultation. The official title for the specialty and its clinics is genitourinary medicine.

People looking after patients with sexually transmitted diseases should use language that is easily understood by the patient, including slang when appropriate. Health care staff may well have different moral and sexual attitudes from their patients. They have to accept and come to terms with this and their own sexuality before being able to cope with patients. It is bad manners for staff to force their own attitudes on a patient and it is also bad medicine, since the patient will not come back.

Contact tracing

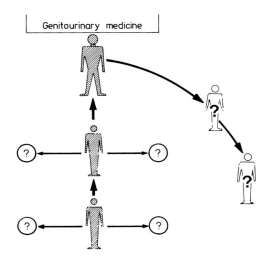

Tracing sexual contacts is an essential part of a control programme. Interviewing patients about their contacts requires tact, sensitivity, and special communication skills. For any one patient (index case) presenting to a clinic there are at least two other people affected—the person who infected the patient and the person who infected that contact. It is usually more complicated than this, so that by the time the index patient has sought medical care he or she may have had intercourse with a further individual. It is essential, therefore, to get in touch as soon as possible with sexual contacts and advise them to attend a clinic. The aim is to control the disease within the community as well as to protect the health of individuals who are symptomless and unaware of their disease. For women with gonococcal and chlamydial infections the prevention of costly disability is of paramount importance.

Some patients feel that being asked about contacts is unnecessary or an infringement of their privacy. The reasons for tracing contacts must be explained to the patient and their active cooperation sought. Often this is a useful health education exercise.

Education and information

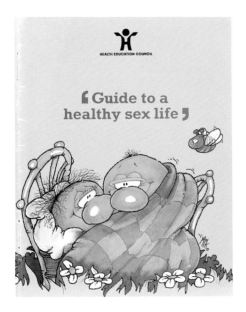

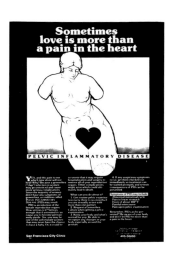

Education of the public and health care workers is an important control measure. Society cannot continue to remain ambivalent about health education for sexually transmitted diseases. There is no evidence that widely available information about these diseases (or about contraception) encourages immoral or promiscuous behaviour.

Primary prevention should aim at educating individuals about the advantages of discriminate and safe sex and prophylaxis. It has to be accepted, however, that there is no agreement in Western society about what constitutes "normal" sexual behaviour. The skilled educator acknowledges this and constructs information that allows an individual, whatever his or her beliefs, to indentify with some, if not all, of what is said. Education about sexually transmitted diseases should cover a wide range of sexual attitudes and behaviour. The best way to avoid sexually transmitted disease is to avoid sexual intercourse. This may not, however, be acceptable to those already sexually active, and they may want to know that monogamous sexual intercourse will cut down the risk. Again, this message may not be acceptable, but it should be pointed out that changing partners often increases greatly the risk of contracting diseases. Awareness of the presenting symptoms of the common diseases is important, but it is also important to point out that disease can be asymptomatic and that regular check ups (every three months) are a wise precaution for those changing their partners often. The use of a barrier contraceptive will reduce the risk of certain diseases and is a wise prophylactic measure when changing sexual partners. The sheath may, however, give a false sense of security.

The importance of the condom has been emphasised in the past few years particularly in relation to HIV infection. Health education can work, as witnessed by a decline in syphilis and gonorrhoea among

---

Reducing the risk of contracting a sexually transmitted disease

(1) Abstain

(2) Avoid multiple partners, prostitutes, and other people with multiple sex partners

(3) Avoid sexual contact with people who have symptoms or lesions (eg urethral discharge, warts, ulcers)

(4) Avoid genital contact with oral "cold sores"

(5) Use condoms or diaphragm

(6) Have regular check ups if at high risk of sexually transmitted disease

Methods of control

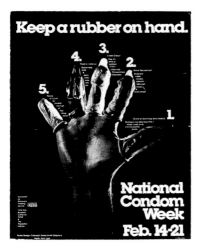

How a patient is managed

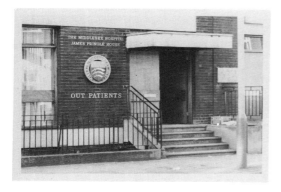

Recorded message (London)
(01) 246-8072

What happens in a clinic

Date of 1st Attendance	THE MIDDLESEX HOSPITAL OUT-PATIENT DEPARTMENT JAMES PRINGLE HOUSE Dr. J.S. BINGHAM Prof. M.W. ADLER	Index No.	
Name		Age	Date of Birth
Address		Civil State	
Occupation		Nationality	
Referred by		District	
History of Present Illness			
Recent Intercourse			
Contacts			
Contraception			
Previous Infections			
Past History			
Family History		Previous Penicillin or Antibiotics Reactions	

homosexual men who have modified their sexual behaviour in the light of the HIV epidemic.

Secondary prevention aims at encouraging people to seek care without delay once the symptoms of a disease are recognised, stop sexual intercourse until medical advice has been sought, and adhere to the advice given.

Since sexually transmitted disease is such a major health problem, more resources need to be devoted towards health education and making the public aware of clinics. Facilities should be advertised in places frequented more readily and openly by the public and not furtively in public toilets. Finally, research should play an important part in the control of the sexually transmitted diseases. Information on the size of the problem, infectivity, aetiology, behavioural determinants, and long term sequelae are central to understanding the diseases as epidemic phenomena, planning appropriate medical and other facilities, and monitoring changes.

Any doctor may refer a patient to a department of genitourinary medicine for diagnosis or treatment or to ensure contact tracing. The earlier chapters have given guidelines on how to recognise and diagnose disease and which patients to refer. Physicians working in departments of genitournary medicine are always happy to see any patient in whom a sexually transmitted disease is suspected or needs to be excluded.

Patients may be extremely anxious about their condition, talking about sexual matters, and what investigations will be performed. Some of these fears can be modified if the person referring the patient can explain how a clinic works.

Finding a clinic—Most patients refer themselves to clinics and often know of a clinic through friends or sexual contacts, or they may be referred by a general practitioner or family planning clinic. Otherwise, information about sexually transmitted disease clinics can be obtained in most large cities from recorded messages and telephone directories. In recent years magazines have printed articles about the sexually transmitted diseases and given star ratings to some clinics and crossed wooden spoons to others. Information of this sort helps patients to find out where the clinics are and the quality of service they may expect.

Some clinics have an appointments system, and a new patient gets an appointment, usually within 24–48 hours, by ringing or visiting the clinic. Other clinics have no appointments and simply invite patients to walk in and be seen. Some run a combined system.

New patients have to register in the clinic. Most clinics have a record system separate from that of the main hospital to ensure confidentiality, and patients do not have to give any personal or demographic details, though few refuse. Then, if laboratory tests are positive and a patient fails to keep an appointment he or she can be told of the results and of the importance of attending. If a patient specifically requests no correspondence, this is respected.

The consultation—Details of the presenting symptoms and their duration are taken and information elicited to exclude possible complications—for example, abdominal pain, arthralgia. Patients will be asked about the occurrence and timing of symptoms in relation to sexual exposure and menstruation, the type of contraception used, the number of recent sexual contacts and whether any of these have symptoms and have received treatment. The sexual orientation of the patient is important. Homosexual patients do not always volunteer this information, particularly if they are under 21 and think that the doctor will report them to the police. If the patient is homosexual he will be asked about the sites put at risk of infection. Finally, a history of previous sexually transmitted disease and sensitivity to antibiotics will be obtained from all patients and, in women, details of any menstrual changes, pregnancies, and recent gynaecological procedures and cervical cytology.

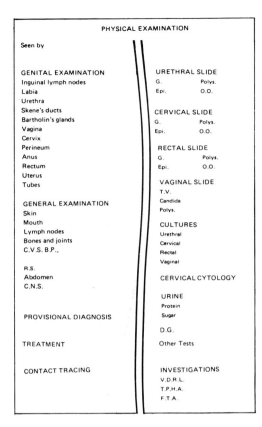

PHYSICAL EXAMINATION

Seen by

GENITAL EXAMINATION
Inguinal lymph nodes
Labia
Urethra
Skene's ducts
Bartholin's glands
Vagina
Cervix
Perineum
Anus
Rectum
Uterus
Tubes

GENERAL EXAMINATION
Skin
Mouth
Lymph nodes
Bones and joints
C.V.S. B.P.,

R.S.
Abdomen
C.N.S.

PROVISIONAL DIAGNOSIS

TREATMENT

CONTACT TRACING

URETHRAL SLIDE
G.   Polys.
Epi.   O.O.

CERVICAL SLIDE
G.   Polys.
Epi.   O.O.

RECTAL SLIDE
G.   Polys.
Epi.   O.O.

VAGINAL SLIDE
T.V.
Candida
Polys.

CULTURES
Urethral
Cervical
Rectal
Vaginal

CERVICAL CYTOLOGY

URINE
Protein
Sugar

D.G.

Other Tests

INVESTIGATIONS
V.D.R.L.
T.P.H.A.
F.T.A.

PLEASE MAKE SURE YOU BRING THIS FORM WITH YOU WHEN YOU ATTEND

HOSPITAL OF ORIGIN:

THE MIDDLESEX HOSPITAL
JAMES PRINGLE HOUSE
73-75 CHARLOTTE STREET
LONDON, W1P 1LB

Telephone Number 01-636 8333
Extension 666
01-323 4819

Mondays to Fridays
9 a.m. — 6.30 p.m.

Dr. J. S. BINGHAM
Prof. M. W. ADLER

APPOINTMENT ADVISED

REF.
No.   DIAGNOSIS
                     (MINISTRY OF HEALTH CODE)
DATE

Confidentiality

Brook Advisory Centres: 233 Tottenham Court Road, London W1. 01-323 1522/580 2991.
2 Lower Gilmore Place, Edinburgh 3. 031-229 5320.
Family Planning Association Information Service: 27 Mortimer Street, London W1. 01-636 7866.
Gay Switchboard: 01-837 7324.
Lesbian Line: 01-251 6911.
Health Education Authority, Mabledon Place, London WC1H 9TX. 01-387 0550.
Scottish Health Education Unit: Woodburn House, Canaan Lane, Edinburgh 10. 031-447 8044.
Hepatitis B Support Group: 01-603 6516/373 6105.
Herpes Association: 41 North Road, London N7. 01-609 9061.
Marriage Guidance Council: 76A New Cavendish Street, London W1. 01-580 1087.
Rape Crisis Centre: PO Box 69, London WC1. 01-837 1600.
PO Box 120, Head Post Office, Edinburgh 1. 031-556 9437.

The examination—A local genital examination is carried out and selectively or routinely augmented by a general physical examination. *Women* are usually examined in the lithotomy position and the external genitalia examined for evidence of disease. Specimens for microscopy and culture are taken from the posterior fornix, vaginal wall, endocervix, and urethra (see chapter on vaginal discharge). Cervical cytology may also be performed. In selected patients proctoscopy is performed and specimens taken (if the patient is a contact of someone with gonorrhoea or volunteers anal or rectal symptoms). This is followed by a bimanual examination. Serological tests for syphilis are performed in all patients since this can be a concurrent asymptomatic infection. Additional tests—haemoglobin, midstream urine, throat swab—are performed if indicated. Finally, urine is tested for protein and sugar. Microscopy can be performed immediately in the clinic and in most cases a diagnosis obtained. If this is not always possible—for example in women—the need to culture specimens is explained and patients are asked to return in three to seven days. In *men* general physical and local genital examinations are performed and samples obtained. Anal examination and proctoscopy and sampling are carried out when indicated. In homosexuals samples are taken from the sites related to the symptoms or, if asymptomatic, from the sites at risk. As in women, serological tests for syphilis, urine tests, and any necessary additional tests are performed. Testing for antibodies to HIV is performed only after counselling and consent.

Treatment—If a sexually transmitted disease is diagnosed microscopically within the clinic the patient will be given treatment at once. All treatment is free of prescription charges.

Contact tracing will be undertaken by contact tracers (social health advisers) or doctors. The social health adviser or patient can visit or telephone contacts. Contact slips are still used, but with the wider availability of telephones they are no longer so popular. A contact slip will be given to the contact(s) by the patient or health adviser. This can be taken to any clinic in the United Kingdom. The slip includes the original patient's note number and a code for the diagnosis. This diagnosis is vital information for the doctor seeing the contact and will help him decide on the appropriate tests. If the contact is seen at a different clinic from the index case the slip will be returned to the original clinic so that accurate contact tracing records can be kept.

The confidentiality of information imparted by patients to doctors or contact tracers is paramount in the practice of genitourinary medicine. Failure to keep confidences will dissuade patients from seeking attention or volunteering information about their sexual orientation and contacts. It is essential that patients should realise that their diagnosis or, indeed, any other information is never given to their sexual partners when they consult or to any one else outside the clinic. Family practitioners are informed of the diagnosis and treatment if the patient has been referred by them in the first instance. Any inquiries, for example from solicitors or doctors performing life assurance examinations, are not answered unless the patient gives written permission. A record keeping system separate from the rest of the hospital secures the confidential nature of information. The police are never given information, even if the patient is a minor, unless the patient requests it.

I am grateful to a number of my colleagues who have commented on this series as it was being written. I am particularly grateful to Drs R S Morton and T Moss, who read and commented on every article. I would also like to thank Dr J S Bingham, Dr G Levene, Dr A Mindel, Dr J D Oriel, Professor C Peckham, Dr G Ridgway, and the late Dr R R Wilcox for their comments on individual articles and the Communicable Disease Surveillance Centre for the use of some of their data. I would like to thank colleagues who have allowed me to use their photographic material (Drs A Attenburrow, J Bingham, and M Waugh) and the photographic department of the Middlesex Hospital Medical school for their help. The illustrations of dark ground microscopy and gonococcal ophthalmia neonatorum were taken from King A, Nicol C, Robin P. *Venereal Diseases*, published by Baillière Tindall. Finally, my secretary Kate Sarra has shown considerable skill, patience, and good humour in typing the articles more often than she might have liked.

Index

Abdominal pain 9, 17, 37, 51
Abortion, spontaneous 57
Acyclovir 26, 38, 58
Africa 32
AIDS 1, 5 *See also* HIV
　definition 32
　epidemiology 32
　gastrointestinal complications 36
　hepatic complications 37
　immunology 33
　natural history 34
　neurological complications 37
　prevention and control 39
　psychiatric symptoms 63
　pulmonary complications 35–6
　related complex 34
　treatment 37, 39
　tumours 34–5
Albumin 29
Alcohol 14, 29, 30
Amoxycillin 7
Amphotericin 38
Ampicillin 7, 18, 19, 20
Anaemia 35, 38
Anaerobic bacteria 11, 18
Anal intercourse 11, 28, 48
Analgesics 26
Aneurysms 52
Anorectum
　carcinoma 35
　herpes 25, 26
Anorexia 50
Antidepressants 61, 62
Antiviral agents 26, 37, 39
Anus 49
　examination 67
　trauma 23
　warts 40, 41
Anxiety 8, 60, 62, 63
Aorta 20, 52, 55
Argyll Robertson pupils 51, 52
Arterial oxygen tension 35
Arthralgia 9
Arthritis 20
Arthropathy 52
Aspirin 55

Bacteraemia 36, 50
Balanitis 22
　candidal 13
　circinate 20, 23
　xerotica obliterans 23, 46
Bartholin's abscess 18
Behaviour changes 37
Behaviour therapy 61
Behçet's disease 22, 23
Benzoic acid compound 45
Benzyl benzoate 44
Benzylpenicillin 7, 18, 58, 60
Blood tests 6, 11
Blood transfusion 29
Bone marrow 35
Bone, syphilitic lesions of 52, 60
Brain 52
　atrophy 37, 51
　blood vessels 51
　damage 57
　necropsy 37
　toxoplasmosis 37, 38
Breath, shortness of 35
Bronchoscopy 35
Buschke-Lowenstein tumour 41

Caesarean section 42, 57–8
Campylobacter 36
Candida albicans 4, 9, 15, 36, 41, 62
　microscopy and culture 10

Candidiasis 1, 10, 38
　empirical treatment 15, 16
　management 13–14
　oesophageal 36
　oral 34, 36
　predisposing factors 13
　psychological problems 62
　recurrence 13
Carbaryl 43
Carbon monoxide transfer factor 35
Carcinoma 23
　cervical 27
　hepatocellular 30
　squamous cell 35, 46
CD4 cells 33, 37
CD4, recombinant 39
Cefoxitin 18
Cefuroxime 8, 18
Central nervous system 37
Cerebrospinal fluid 37, 54, 55
Cervical intraepithelial neoplasia 41
Cervix uteri 11, 18
　cytology 11, 26, 27, 67
　herpes 25, 26, 27
　lesions 9, 49, 50
　neoplasms 27
　warts 40, 41
Chancroid 22, 23
Charcot's arthropathy 52
Chest
　discomfort 35, 36
　pain 52
　x rays 35, 55, 58
Child abuse 63
Chlamydia trachomatis 4, 5, 7, 8, 9, 11,
　　17, 18, 20, 41
　antigen detection 6
Chlamydial infections 5, 7, 8, 15, 18, 26
　incubation period 4
　neonatal 58
Cholangitis 37
Cholecystitis 37
Cholestasis 29
Cirrhosis of liver 30
Clindamycin 18
Ciprofloxacin 7, 20
Climate 25
Clindamycin 38
Clinics *See* Departments of genitourinary
　　medicine
Clotrimazole 13, 45
Co-trimoxazole 7, 18, 20, 26, 38
Coal tar 47
Coma 14
Computed tomography 35, 37
Condoms 27, 65
Condylomata acuminata *See* Genital warts
Condylomata lata 50
Confidentiality 67
Conjunctivitis 20, 58
Constipation 25
Contact tracing 3, 5, 8, 14, 15, 18, 19, 20,
　　41, 65
　candidiasis 13
　hepatitis 31
　method 67
　scabies 44
　syphilis 55
Contraceptives
　barrier 65
　intrauterine 2, 9, 17
　oral 2, 9
Corticosteroid cream 46, 47
Cough 35, 52
Counselling 1
　herpes 27
　HIV antibody testing 62–3, 67

rape victims 63
　under aged 63
Cranial nerve palsies 51
Cryotherapy 41, 42
Cryptococcosis 38
Cryptosporidium 36, 37
　infections 38
Culture 67
　C albicans 10
　fungi 45
　herpes 26
　N gonorrhoeae 5, 10
Cystitis 6
Cytomegalovirus 1, 28, 29, 36, 37
　treatment 38, 39

Dapsone 38
Delusions 61
Dementia 37, 51, 63
Departments of genitourinary medicine 1,
　　64
　confidentiality 67
　consultation 66
　contact tracing 67
　examination 67
　finding a clinic 66
　referral 3, 7, 66
　routine tests 10
　treatment 67
Depression 19, 62, 63
Dermatitis 22, 47
　artefacta 4, 23, 48
Diarrhoea 34, 36
2'3' Dideoxycytidine 38
2'3' Dideoxyinosine 38
Doxycycline 7, 8, 18, 19
Drugs 29, 37
　absorption 14
　eruptions 22
　See also Intravenous drug abuse
Dyspareunia 9, 17, 46, 62
Dysphagia 36, 52
Dysuria 19

Econazole 45
Education *See* Health education
Electrocautery 41, 42
Encephalitis 37
　herpes 58
Encephalopathy, HIV 37, 63
Enteric pathogens 1
Enteropathy 36
Eosinophilia 58
Epidermophyton floccosum 45
Epididymitis 19
Epstein-Barr virus 28, 29
Erythema multiforme 22
Erythromycin 8, 18, 19, 38, 55, 58
　placental transfer 59
Eyes
　congenital syphilis 60
　neonatal infections 58–9

Face 42
　congenital syphilis 60
False positive reactions 54
Fatigue 29, 35, 63
Feet 20
　soles 5
　ulcers 52
Fetus 27
　death 57
　syphilis 59
Fever 19, 25, 29, 34, 35, 36, 37, 50, 55
Fluconazole 38, 39
Flucytosine 38

Fluorescent treponemal antibody (FTA) test 54, 60
Folliculitis 22, 34
Furuncles 22

Gamma benzene hexachloride 43, 44
Ganciclovir 38, 39
Garnerella vaginalis 9, 11, 41
Gastrointestinal tract
  AIDS 34, 35, 36
  gummas 52
General paralysis of the insane 51
Genital examination 5, 67
Genital ulcers
  diagnosis 23
  multiple painful 22
  solitary painless 23
Genital warts 4, 9
  clinical features 41
  complications 41
  diagnosis 41
  increase 1
  incubation 40
  treatment 41–2
  virus 41
Genitourinary medicine 3
  See also Departments of genitourinary
    medicine
Gentamicin 18
Gonococcal infections
  disseminated 20
  neonatal 58–9
  See also Gonorrhoea
Gonococcal urethritis
  chemotherapy 7
  follow up 8
  psychological problems 62
  treatment failure 8
Gonococcus *See Neisseria gonorrhoeae*
Gonorrhoea 5, 18, 19, 26, 41
  incidence 1, 64
  incubation period 4
  oropharyngeal 20
  rectal 20, 41
Granuloma inguinale 23
Griseofulvin 45
Groins 47
  pain 25
  rash 45

Haemophilia 28
Haemophilus ducreyi 22
Haemospermia 19
Hands 20
Headaches 25, 29, 51
Health care staff
  attitude of 64
  education 65
Health education 39, 65–6
Hearing impairment 60
Heart block 20
Hepatitis 28–31, 37
Hepatitis A 1, 28, 31
  diagnosis 29
  virus 28
Hepatitis B 1
  antibodies and antigens 29, 30, 31
  chronic infection 30
  groups at risk 28
  HIV infection 31
  sexual contacts 31
  vaccine 31
  virus 28
Hepatitis D 30
  virus 28
Hepatitis, non-A, non-B
  chronic infection 30
  serological diagnosis 29
  viruses 28
  waterborne epidemics 28

Hepatitis, viral
  causes 28
  clinical features 29
  complications 30
  fulminant 28, 30
  history 29
  hospital admission 30
  incubation 28
  laboratory tests 29
  management 30
  prevention 31
  serological tests 29
  transmission 28
Hepatocellular carcinoma 30
Herpes Association 27
Herpes simplex infections 4, 9 23, 34, 38
  anorectal 25
  antiviral agents 26
  asymptomatic 25
  counselling 27
  diagnosis 26
  incidence 1, 24
  pregnancy and neonatal 57–8
  primary 25
  psychiatric illness 62
  recurrent 25, 62
  routine management 26
  Type 1 24
  Type 2 25, 27
  vaccine 27
Herpes simplex virus 22, 36, 37
  antibodies 24
  classification 24
  culture 26
  shedding 26, 27
  transmission 24
Herpes zoster 34
HIV *See also* HIV infection
  antibody testing 34, 62, 67
  encephalopathy 37
  properties 33
  transmission 32
HIV infection 5
  acute 34
  adjustment reaction 63
  chronic 34
  classification 34
  counselling 62, 67
  hepatitis B 31
  progression to AIDS 34
  serological profile 33
Homosexual men 5, 20, 26, 41, 66, 67
  AIDS 32, 34, 35
  HIV infected 62
  syphilis 1, 49
Human immunodeficiency virus *See* HIV
Human papillomavirus 35, 40, 41
Hydrocortisone 48
Hypnotherapy 62
Hypochondriasis 61, 63
Hypokalaemia 41

Ice packs 26
Idoxuridine 26
IgG antibodies 29, 33, 58
IgM antibodies 29, 33, 58, 60
Imidazoles 13, 45
Immune dysfunction 33
Impetigo 22, 34
Impotence 19
Indomethacin 20
Infections
  concurrent 10, 11, 13, 14, 15, 31
  local complications 17–9
  opportunistic 34, 35–7, 38
  systemic complications 20
Infertility 17, 62
Infestations 43–5
Interferon, alfa 30, 39
Interferon, gamma 33
Intravenous drug abuse 28, 29, 32, 62

Isospora belli 36
  infections 38

Jarisch-Herxheimer reaction 55
Jaundice 29
Joints 5, 20
  Clutton's 60
  tabes dorsalis 52

Kaposi's sarcoma 1, 34–5, 39
Ketoconazole 14, 38

Lactation 14, 43
Larynx 50, 52
  papillomas 40, 42
Libido 19
Lichen planus 22, 47
Lichen sclerosus et atrophicus 46
Liver 52
  biopsy 30
  cirrhosis 30
  disease 28, 30
  enlarged 37
  failure 30
  function tests 29, 30, 37
  infections in AIDS 37
  see also Hepatitis
Lungs 35–6, 52
Lymph nodes
  axillary 34
  cervical 34
  inguinal 22, 23, 25, 49
Lymphadenopathy 34, 50
Lymphocele 48
Lymphocytes, CD4 37
Lymphocytic interstitial pneumonitis 36
Lymphogranuloma venereum 23

Malabsorption 36
Malaise 25, 34, 35, 50
Malathion 43, 44
Marital problems 63
Meningitis 25, 26, 37, 51
Meningoencephalitis 20, 34, 37, 51
Meningomyelitis 25
Menstruation 9, 17, 25
Metronidazole 14, 15, 18
Miconazole 38, 45
Microscopy 5, 8, 10, 15, 19, 67
  dark ground 53
Micturition, frequency 19
Milk products 8
Minocycline 19
Molluscum contagiosum 42
Mouth 5, 20, 50
  candidiasis 34
  carcinoma 35
  congenital syphilis 60
  gummas 52
  leukoplakia 34
  ulcers 22
Myalgia 34
Mycobacteria 36, 37
Mycobacterium tuberculosis 36
Myelopathy 37
Myopathy 37

Nails 20, 47
Nasal septum 52, 60
Neisseria gonorrhoeae 4, 7, 9, 11, 17, 20, 41
  culture 5, 10
  penicillin resistant strains 2, 5, 8, 18
Neonate 27
  chlamydial infections 58
  gonococcal infections 58–9
  herpes 57–8
  laryngeal papillomas 40, 42
  syphilis 59–60
Nephritis 4, 6

Neuropathies 37
    peripheral 20, 37, 39, 41
Neurosyphilis 51–2
    changes in cerebrospinal fluid 55
    lumbar puncture 54
    prognosis and treatment 55
Neutropenia 38
Night sweats 34, 35
Nimorazole 14
Non-gonococcal urethritis 4, 20, 41
    chemotherapy 8
    follow up 8
    microscopy 5
    psychological problems 62
Non-Hodgkin's lymphoma 35
Non-steriodal anti-inflammatory agents 20
Nose 50, 60
Nystatin 13, 38

Oesophagus
    candidiasis 36
Ophthalmia neonatorum 58
Opportunistic infections 34, 35–7
    treatment 38
Oral hairy leukoplakia 34
Orchitis 19
Otitis media 58
Oxytetracycline 7, 8

Pain
    chest 52
    herpes 25, 26
    pelvic 62
    penis 46, 48
    prostatitis 19, 62
Patient
    anxious 8
    compliance 8, 13, 14
    sexual orientation 5, 66
Pediculosis pubis 43
Pelvic inflammatory disease
    costs 64
    diagnosis 17
    morbidity 17
    psychological problems 62
    treatment 18, 21
Penicillin 7, 8, 15, 18, 19, 20, 58
    gonococcal resistance 2, 5, 8, 18
    syphilis 55, 59
Penis 4, 9, 20, 22, 44, 47, 50
    bending 48
    examination 5
    pain 46, 48
    trauma 23
    warts 40, 41
Pentamidine 38, 39
Perianal area 5, 47
Pericarditis 20
Perineum 40, 47
Peyronie's disease 48
Pharyngitis 34
Pharynx 50, 52, 58
Phenol 42
Phimosis 46
Phobias 1, 61
Phosphonoformate 39
Photophobia 25
Phthirue pubis 43
Pneumocystis carinii pneumonia
    presentation and diagnosis 35
    treatment 38–9
Pneumonia
    bacterial 36
    chlamydial 58
    P carinii 35, 38, 39
Podophyllin 41, 42
Podophyllotoxin 41
Pregnancy 14, 43
    genital warts 41, 42
    herpes 57–8

syphilis 59
    tubal 17
Probenecid 7, 8, 18, 19, 20
Procaine penicillin 7, 18, 55, 59, 60
Proctitis 11
Proctoscopy 41, 67
Prostate gland 19
Prostatitis 19, 62
Prostatorrhoea 4
Prothrombin time 29
Protozoal infections 36, 38
Pruritis vulvae 46
Psoriasis 22, 47
Psychiatric disease
    primary 61
    secondary to STD 62–3
Psychological sequelae
    AIDS 63
    genital lesions 48, 62
    HIV infection 62
    pelvic inflammatory disease 17, 62
    syphilis 62
Psychosexual problems 63
Pubic hair 5
Pubic louse 43
Pyrimethamine 38
Pyuria 8

Rape victims 63
Rapid plasma reagin (RPR) test 53
Rash 9, 34, 44
    tinea cruris 45
Rectum 5, 11, 40, 49, 58
    discharge 25
    gonorrhoea 20, 41
    trauma 23, 48
Reiter's disease 20, 22
Respiratory system ·35–6
Retroviruses 33

Sadomasochism 23, 48
Salmonella 20, 36
Salpingitis 17, 18
Salt baths 26
Sarcoptes scabiei 44
Scabies 1, 22, 23
    diagnosis and treatment 44–5
    mite 44
    symptoms 44
Scrotum 5, 40, 44, 47
    support 19
Seborrhoeic dermatitis 34
Self examination 8
Self inflicted trauma 4, 22, 23, 47, 48
Self medication 4
Serological tests
    hepatitis 29
    syphilis 53–4, 60, 67
Sexual aids 4, 9, 48
Sexual contacts See Contact tracing
Sexual intercourse 2, 4, 8, 11, 13, 22, 24,
        25, 27
    HIV transmission 32
    psychosocial factors 61
Sexually transmitted diseases
    addresses 67
    cases in United Kingdom 3
    clinics 64, 66–7
    contact tracing 65, 67
    increase 1, 2, 64
    information 66
    management 3
    micro-organisms 3
    presentation 2
    risk reduction 65
    secondary psychiatric disease 62–3
    variety 1
Shigella 20
Skin 5
    conditions 34, 46–7
    lesions 25, 49–50, 52

"Snail track" ulcers 50
Spectinomycin 7, 8, 18
Spermatorrhoea 4
Spermatozoa 11
Spinal cord 51
Spiramycin 38
Sterility 17
Steroids 55
Stevens-Johnson syndrome 22
Streptococci, β-haemolytic 1, 9, 22
Stress 25
Sulfadoxine 38
Sulphadiazine 38
Syphilis 4, 6, 7, 8, 9, 11, 23, 26, 41, 43
    cardiovascular 51, 52, 55
    cerebrospinal fluid 54–5
    congenital 59–60, 62
    dark ground microscopy 53
    extent of the problem 49, 64
    gummatous 51, 52
    incidence 1, 49
    latent 51
    meningovascular disease 51
    parenchymatous neurosyphilis 51–2
    pregnancy 59
    primary 49
    prognosis 55
    psychological problems 62
    radiology 55
    secondary 49
    serological tests 53–4, 67
    treatment 55, 56

Tabes dorsalis 51–2
Tattoos 29
Teeth 60
Teratogenesis 14
Testes 19, 52
Tetracycline 7, 8, 15, 18, 19, 20, 55
Throat 5
    gonorrhoea 20
Tinea crusis 45
Tinea infections 34
Torulopsis glabrata 10
Toxic shock syndrome 9
Toxoplasmosis 37, 38
Trauma, genital 4, 9, 13, 48
Treponema pallidum
    haemagglutination test (TPHA) 54, 60
    identification 53
    placental transfer 59
Trichloroacetic (trichloroethanoic)
        acid 41, 42
Trichomonas vaginalis 4, 5, 9, 11, 14, 41
    microscopy 10
Trichomoniasis 10, 26
    management 14
    psychological problems 62
Trichophyton rubrum 45
Tuberculosis, pulmonary 36
Tumours in AIDS 34–5

Ulceration
    feet 52
    genital–22–3
    gut 36
Ureaplasma urealyticum 4, 9
Urethra 5, 14, 40
    female 11, 18
    meatal narrowing 46
    trauma 4
Urethral discharge 19, 46
    blood and urine tests 6
    causes 4
    clinical features 4–5
    culture 5–6
    management 7–8
    microscopy 5, 8
    physical examination 5
    referral 7
    sexual factors 5

Urethritis
  anterior 6
  asymptomatic 5
  gonococcal 7–8, 62
  non-gonococcal 4, 5, 8, 20, 62
  posterior 6, 19
  postgonococcal 8
Urinary tract infections 4, 19
Urine
  obstruction 46
  retention 25, 26
  tests 6, 11, 67
Uveitis 20

Vagina 10, 40, 46, 50
  bacteria 14

retained products 9
  trauma 9, 13
Vaginal discharge
  causes 9
  fishy odour 11, 62
  high risk profile 9, 15
  history 9–10
  investigations 10–12
  management by non-specialist 15
  treatment 13, 14, 15
Vaginismus 62
Vaginitis, non-specific *See* Vaginosis,
    anaerobic
Vaginosis, anaerobic 11, 62
  treatment 15
Venereal Disease Research Laboratory

(VDRL) test 53, 54, 60
Vidarabine 58
Vincent's organisms 22
Viral hepatitis *See* Hepatitis
Vulva 18, 25, 26, 47, 50
  irritation 13, 15, 46
  warts 40, 41
Vulvitis 22

Warts *See* Genital warts
Weight loss 34, 35, 36
Whitfield's ointment 45

Yersinia 20

Zidovudine 37, 39